HUMAN CENTERED NURSING

The Foundation of Quality Care

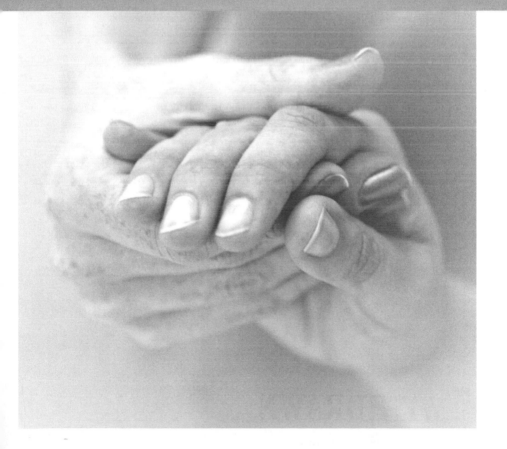

HUMAN CENTERED NURSING

The Foundation of Quality Care

By
Susan Kleiman, PhD, RN, CS, NPP

Founder, International Institute for Human Centered Caring
Assistant Professor of Nursing and
Director of Graduate Studies in Nursing
Professor of Qualitative Research for the Graduate Center,
City University of New York Doctoral Program in Nursing

F. A. Davis Company
1915 Arch Street
Philadelphia, PA 19103
www.fadavis.com

Printed in the United States of America

Last digit indicates print number: 1 9 8 7 6 5 4 3 2 1

Publisher, Nursing: Joanne P. DaCunha, RN, MSN
Director of Content Development: Darlene D. Pedersen
Development Editor: Kristin L. Kern
Manager of Art & Design: Carolyn O'Brien

As new scientific information becomes available through basic and clinical research, recommended treatments and drug therapies undergo changes. The author(s) and publisher have done everything possible to make this book accurate, up to date, and in accord with accepted standards at the time of publication. The author(s), editors, and publisher are not responsible for errors or omissions or for consequences from application of the book, and make no warranty, expressed or implied, in regard to the contents of the book. Any practice described in this book should be applied by the reader in accordance with professional standards of care used in regard to the unique circumstances that may apply in each situation. The reader is advised always to check product information (package inserts) for changes and new information regarding dose and contraindications before administering any drug. Caution is especially urged when using new or infrequently ordered drugs.

Library of Congress Cataloging-in-Publication Data

Kleiman, Susan.
 Human centered nursing : the foundation of quality care / by Susan Kleiman.
   p. ; cm.
 Includes bibliographical references.
 ISBN 978-0-8036-1485-7 (pbk. : alk. paper)
 1. Nurse and patient. 2. Nursing–Philosophy. 3. Humanism. I. Title.
 [DNLM: 1. Humanism. 2. Nurse-Patient Relations–ethics. 3. Nursing Care–methods. 4. Patient-Centered Care. 5. Philosophy, Nursing. WY 87 K63h 2009]
 RT86.3.K64 2009
 610.73–dc22

                                                        2008005132

Preface

A s we engage in the fast-paced and complex activities of daily nursing, we can forget the essential nature of the human centered enterprise in which we are engaged. Some of the most beautiful and tragic of life's experiences come to nurses through the intimate relationships we form as we take part in the lives of our patients, their families, students, and other health-care professionals.

In this book I show a way to look beyond the daily hustle and bustle of a busy health-care setting in order to reflect on what it truly means to be a nurse, both in a professional and a personal sense. The book is about the reality of nursing. Although it is written for nursing students, it will also resonate with teachers, practicing nurses, and those interested in nursing or becoming a nurse. Little time is spent on "what" it is that nurses "do" as there are many fine texts available on those subjects. Instead, the emphasis is on the "why" of nursing practice and how nurses' lives are changed and enriched by those they touch and those who touch them.

Perhaps one reader will relate to one or more of the experiences described and uncover his own meanings and values hidden within it. Perhaps another reader will be inspired to share her own values, beliefs, and life experiences. Perhaps yet another reader will gain an awareness of the possibilities that sharing, being with, and doing with others hold for each of us to become more as human beings. I hope that all readers will be encouraged to find their voice and be able to articulate what it is they have come to know with confidence and pride.

After all is said and done, the purpose of this book is to reemphasize the essence of the nursing act as it is articulated in the Human Centered Nursing Model. Human centered nursing practice is the foundation of high-quality patient care; it is the model that supports the acquisition of practical skills necessary for competent and ethically grounded nursing practice. Quality patient care is presented within the context of everyday influences such as culture and professional core beliefs and values, including the Nurses' Code of Ethics (2001) and Nursing's Social Policy

Statement (2003). These are intended to instill a sense of professional authority and add substance and strength to nursing's professional voice.

This book is a composition about human centered nursing and its foundational concepts and essential qualities, which appear in various juxtapositions and evolve under different moments of nursing occasions. These human centered nursing moments are marked by the awareness of the uniqueness of the individual and the affirmation of the "I–Thou" mode of being-with others.

The style of presentation is intended to invigorate and actualize the readers' potential for learning. The method is one of learning to learn through thinking. The kind of thinking I am proposing is less exact than the familiar calculative and deductive type associated with problem solving and the technical and technological aspects of nursing; it is a more expansive and inquisitive type through which we seek the essential nature of something—the affirmation of learning.

In this schema, the function of the teacher is to guide the student in the process of learning by way of thinking to help that student bring forward the essential nature of the object of investigation. Heidegger (1993) denotes this style of participation in learning as "to let learn." Accordingly, the proper function of teaching is to open a space for learning, that is, to let-learn.

How does this resonate in the nursing experience? The nurse's main concern is not learning how to use the stethoscope, thermometer, or blood pressure device or how to give an injection or calculate a medication dosage, although these are necessary to the nursing act. Rather, the nurse is primarily concerned with bringing forth the essence of nursing. The student nurse affirms her learning by bringing out the beauty of her nursing project in its essential form, which is participating with patients, families, students, and colleagues, in a process of being and becoming, regardless of the situation in which they find themselves.

I offer many real-life experiences in the book, some my own and others from my students and nurses I have known. The experiences are unedited in order to retain their originality and are offered with the understanding that the meanings of many nursing experiences may be ineffable and un-sayable within the limitations of language.

The inspiration for this book came into being over 25 years ago when I first met nurse educators and theorists Josephine Paterson and Loretta Zderad during a preceptorship. They introduced me to a way of thinking about nursing that I have carried with me through all the phases of my nursing career.

Paterson and Zderad saw the turmoil in the health-care institution, especially as it involved nurses, and offered a way to make things better for nurses. They offered a way of thinking about nursing that would illuminate the beautiful moments that nurses share and value with their patients and loved ones and helped nurses find their voice so they could share those moments with others. Notwithstanding the ever-present confusion and dissatisfaction in the health-care milieu, Paterson and Zderad hoped that nurses would not give up their efforts to help people become all they could be regardless of the situation in which they found themselves and then realize the peaceful self-awareness that comes with being a nurse who has made a difference in the life of another.

This book is my offering to join in Paterson and Zderad's dream for nursing. I invite all other nurses to be and become with me.

REFERENCES

American Nurses Association. (2001). *Nurses code of ethics with interpretive statements.* Nursesbooks.org, Silver Spring, MD.

American Nurses Association. (2003). *Nursing's social policy statement.* Nursesbooks.org, Silver Spring, MD.

Heidegger, M. (1993). *Basic writings,* Ed D. Farrell Krell. San Francisco: Harper.

Reviewers

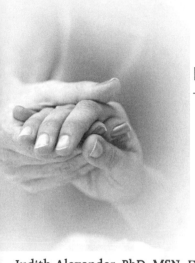

Judith Alexander, PhD, MSN, DNS
Associate Professor
Armstrong Atlantic State University
Savannah, Georgia

Carol Boswell, RN, EdD
Associate Professor
Texas Tech University Health Science
Center
Odessa, Texas

Beverly J.D. Bye, MS, CRNP, FNE-A
Course Coordinator for Childbearing
Families
Towson University
Towson, Maryland

Traudel B. Cline, RN, MSN
Nursing Instructor
Milwaukee Area Technical College
Milwaukee, Wisconsin

Sally E. Erdel, RN, MS
Assistant Professor
Bethel College
Mishawaka, Indiana

Pamela Stewart Fahs, RN, DSN
Associate Professor
Director of the O'Connor Office of Rural
Health Sciences
Binghamton University
Decker School of Nursing
Binghamton, New York

Joyce J. Fitzpatrick, PhD, MBA, FAAN,
FNAP
Professor
Case Western Reserve University
Bolton School of Nursing
Cleveland, Ohio

Linda Ann Kucher, RN, MSN
Assistant Professor
Gordon College
Barnesville, Georgia

Diana M.I. Newman, EdD, RN
Associate Professor
University of Massachusetts
Boston, Massachusetts

Cynthia D. Softhauser, PhD, RN, HNC
Associate Professor
Indiana University
South Bend, Indiana

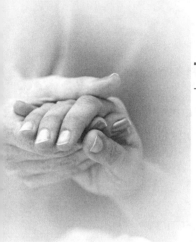

Table of Contents

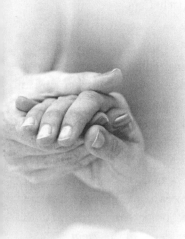

Chapter 1

Introduction to Human Centered Nursing

Walking through the halls of a hospital, nursing home, clinic, or other health/medical care institution, many sounds are heard. These sounds include phones ringing, call bells sounding, meal trays rattling, equipment being pushed about, computers clicking and beeping, and staff being paged. These make up a collage of sounds familiar to the people who work in these settings. These may be called, for lack of a more convenient name, "The Sounds of Health Care."

Other, more subtle, sounds make up this collage as well—such as murmurs of pain, sorrow, anxiety, laughter, joy, or desperation; even silence—that express the state-of-being of the patients. Unlike the familiar sounds that signal the arrival of some form of "equipment," these more subtle sounds are always present and can be "felt," even when they fall outside of the audible range of the human ear. It is as if they are awaiting amplification, ready to be transmitted by some mystical force to those who would hear them. When they come to awareness, they demand immediate attention and sort of "overwhelm" the surrounding sounds of the environment, directing our attention to someone who is calling out for the human touch of a nurse. Take, for example, the cry of a mother: "Where is my baby? What happened to my baby? What's wrong with my baby?"

The call for the human touch of a nurse intensifies and brings into nurses' awareness their own inner calling to offer the human touch that will allow them to experience themselves as nurses. These calls, from one person to another, present possibilities for occasions of human centered nursing, nursing occasions within which nurses respond to patients' calls for help with health-related concerns in a manner that will help patients or their loved ones be as much as they can be in the situation. Helping each person be as much as he or she can be in a given situation, whether that be in birth, death, sickness, disability, dying, or health, is the primary motivation and activity of human centered nursing.

1

In today's health-care milieu there is a resounding call for nurses to reemphasize their humanistic nature, which has been pushed into the background of consciousness by a techno-worship medical model. There is a resounding call to bring the truth of a human-centered nursing experience back into the foreground of thinking and conversations about nursing practice. The call is to reestablish and re-prioritize a human centered nursing motif on behalf of persons seeking health-care services. The call comes most clearly from those nurses who provide direct service to patients. It has long been, after all, the nurse who has provided a competent, professional, and human interface among technology, medicine, and the patient. It is a nurse who participates in the lived experience of the event.

Similarly, there is a call from nursing students who can be overwhelmed by the complexity and magnitude of the scientific/technological imperative given priority in schools of nursing. This imperative prevails despite the fact that nursing students are told over and over again that everything they learn is concerned with doing for and with the patient.

Nursing students, on their first day of class, are introduced to the maxim that nursing is a service profession responsible to society to provide competent, skilled, and humane care (ANA, 2003). This maxim is echoed in nurse practice acts, codes of ethics, social policy statements, and standards of practice, all of which focus on nurses' obligations to provide competent patient care and attend to patients' health-care needs. From this starting point, schools of nursing provide many learning activities that are, of necessity, fact- and skill-oriented: learning parameters of normal values; identifying and describing signs and symptoms; calculating or verifying medication dosages; and acquiring skills such as taking blood pressure, giving injections, doing sterile dressings, suctioning, and catheterizing. Supplementary to the nursing curricula are lessons in interpersonal and communications skills. These are intended, in large part, to give students the ability to collect health histories, obtain physical examination data, and collect other information necessary to the nursing process in order to formulate a care plan.

Upon completion of the formal education process, licensing, and entry into practice, nurses are offered numerous professional and continuing education opportunities for them to maintain skills and to meet the requirements of certification. Again, the emphasis and orientation are on the acquisition of technical skills and competencies.

Despite extensive education in these areas, many of the services that nurses provide for patients cannot be explained in terms of scientific, technological, and mechanical interventions. There are no predefined responses for those unique and unpredictable events that happen at some moment in time, attended to by nurses, patients, and families together. Nurses talk of these moments—handing a newborn to her mother for the very first time, waking a patient who has just had a leg amputation, telling a person that a loved one has died. Because of the unpredictability of nursing, many students, in their first clinical experiences, find themselves unprepared for situations that were never discussed in class or clinic. In fact, there is no way of knowing what will happen at any given moment in the life-world of a nurse.

Keep in mind that as human beings seeking and giving health care, we each are more than an attachment to some form of technological or medical artifice. It is this "more-ness" that is the focal point of human centered nursing. A human centered way of thinking is not contrary to a scientific or technological mode of practice. It is, rather, a complement, augmentation, and clarification of purpose. Think of a coin. Neither side can exist without the other. Metaphorically speaking, each side effectively illuminates aspects or points of view of the central theme of the other. This metaphor helps us understand how the human centered nursing experience harmonizes and is interdependent with the technological and scientific aspects of nursing practice and nursing education. It also explains that each side is necessary to high-quality nursing care and professional satisfaction.

Professional organizations and outside monitoring agencies have taken positions on the professional image and real nature of nursing, issuing mandates that nurses must continue to meet the needs of patients for humanistic care. For example, the American Nurses Association cites in the Code of Ethics for Nurses (2001) (see Appendix B) the importance placed on the nurse's relationship and responsibility to the individual as a human being: "The nurse, in all professional relationships, practices with compassion and respect for the inherent dignity, worth and uniqueness of every individual, unrestricted by considerations of social or economic status, personal attributes, or the nature of health problems" (p. 4).

In a document entitled, "A Vision for Nursing Education" (a collective reflection of the ideas and values of the members and Board of Governors of the National League for Nursing [NLN] developed and published in 1993 and reaffirmed in 2001), caring and humanitarianism are cited core values, not the exclusive use of technology. The NLN document states that "faculty are urgently needed who are prepared to engage in research that will support and advance models that collapse the boundaries between education and practice, professional and patient, and those separating disciplines" (NLN, 2005).

Sigma Theta Tau International, the Honor Society of Nursing (STTI, 2003), in a statement entitled, "The Heart of Nursing," talks about the nature of nurses' work as: "[I]nvolving an exploration of the meanings and values surrounding health, illness, death and dying. . . . Often it is the richness of the interactions that offers nurses their most memorable experiences as they care for those who are undergoing health-threatening challenges. . . . These experiences of interactions with patients, families, and other nurses, enhance nurses' presence and contribute to personal and professional growth."

The National Council Licensure Examination Test Plan for registered nurses (2004) also points out the importance of humanistic aspects of nursing practice, including interpersonal communication; religious and spiritual influences on health; cultural diversity; ethical practice; patients' rights; and universal phenomena, such as illness, wellness, comfort, grief, loss, and caring.

All of these issues highlighted as relevant to good nursing practice are discussed in this book. The following chapters explore these overriding questions:

- How do nurses learn to enhance and value the human centered aspects of patient care?
- How do nurses learn to provide the necessary response to the health-related needs of the patient in a humanistic manner?
- How did nurses' professional ethics evolve from the precepts of human centered care?
- How do nurses learn to value nursing experiences and attain the satisfaction they need to sustain their careers?
- How do nurses integrate and emphasize the human centered nursing approach in daily practice?

REFERENCES

American Nurses Association. (2001). *Code of ethics for nurses with interpretive statements.* Silver Spring, MD.

American Nurses Association. (2003). *Nursing's social policy statement* (2nd Ed.). Washington, DC.

National League for Nursing. (2005). *A vision for nursing.* [on-line]. Available: http://www.nln.org/aboutnln/vision.htm

Paterson, J. & Zderad, L. (1976). *Humanistic nursing.* New York: John Wiley & Sons.

Sigma Theta Tau International. (2003). "Heart of Nursing." [on-line]. Available: www.nursingsociety.org

Permissions

Excerpts used in this chapter from Kleiman, S. (2007). Revitalizing the humanistic imperative in nursing education. *Nursing Education Perspectives* 28(4), 209–213. By permission of the National League for Nursing.

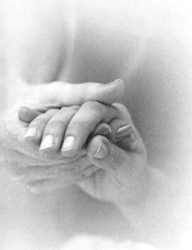

Chapter 2

What is Human Centered Nursing?

Human centered nursing is a lived dialogue, a call-and-response event that occurs between a nurse and a person who come together in a nursing occasion. The impetus for coming together is a health-related concern within which nurses fulfill their professional commitment to provide patient care. The dynamic of coming together and attending to health-related concerns of patients is usually seen, at first glance, as an act of nurturing.

In its simplest form, nurturing is represented by the mother who holds her child in her arms. Incidental to the act of nurturing is the mother's awareness of and response to the concerns of the child. For example, if the child is fearful of the mother's leaving, the mother will nurture the child with physical and verbal reassurance. In this sense, nurturing involves a process between individuals that supports survival and fosters human potential. Within the interchange of the nurturing relationship, mother and child call out to each other, longing to be recognized, each offering to the other the gift of presence that allows them to be and that affirms their existence in the world (Buber, 1965). The offering of the gift of presence is implied, and often concealed, in the act of nurturing.

Presence

Like other gifts, the gift of presence is wrapped in particular, objective outer layers that conceal its true nature and value. Suppose you receive a family heirloom, a chess set. Along with the kings, knights, and pawns, the essence at the heart of this gift is the continuity of family, values, and traditions, handed down from one generation to another. The chess pieces, board, and game-playing skills are the wrappings that conceal the true essence of the gift.

As with other gifts, the gift of presence in nursing may be disguised by the amazing ways in which nurses use their skills to employ the necessary techniques of patient care in performing their duties. Nurses use the tools of the profession

5

within a context that affirms patients as subjective beings like themselves, rather than objects of disease or illness to be acted upon. It is within this context that there arises the possibility for the gift of presence through which a nurse may actualize the value and meaning of nursing.

Presence is not just a mere "being there," nor is it a simple "being at" at a particular time, e.g., being in the same room or checking the reading on some kind of vitals-monitoring equipment. It is rather a being-there-for and a being-there-with, one person directing his or her full attention to another—joining in a life's experience of despair, uncertainty, joy, or as is the case in nursing, a health-related concern—seeing and being seen.

Giving or receiving the gift of presence is similar to experiencing a great work of art in that each occasion is a one-of-a-kind creative interpretation of a nurse's way of being with patients at moments in their life's histories. Furthermore, involvement with a patient, family, colleague, or student is similar to experiencing a work of art in that it evokes an emotional response in the participants.

The experience of giving and receiving the gift of presence is a phenomenon that occurs between two people who are, metaphorically speaking, going through life together. Because each experience that we have becomes a part of who we are, the gift of presence enriches our self-hood; that is, it adds to our life world sets of meanings and values that define us as persons as well as augmenting our recollectible lived-experiences, which we use to guide our actions and ground our motives in future nursing occasions.

Presence fosters connections that extend over time and convey a sense of constancy in nurse-patient relationships. One nurse tells the patients, "I am here, I am still here, I will be here" to reveal dependability and availability and the companionship-like bond between nurse and patient. This connection over time, be it for a day, a week, or longer, differentiates this relationship from the patient's relationship with other health-care professionals who do not offer the same level of involvement or availability.

We often find examples of this phenomenon between patients and nurses. A nurse on a vascular unit talks about working with patients with chronically deteriorating conditions:

> Then I saw her and you know she had a smile on her face, "Oh, you're here," and touched my hand. I said, "I'm still here, anything you need just let me know, I'm here." That's very nice in spite of the fact that it's a very difficult situation, her condition. The fact that you know that their

mind is at peace just because they know you are there when they come to the floor. That's one good thing. Even if you make a difference in only one person's life for the day or the month, it really makes you feel good. I'm sure she's going to remember me for a while, for a long time.

Another nurse recalls offering the gift of presence to a dying boy, unsure of his ability to receive it or recognize it. The lingering and profound impact that the experience of true presence can have on a nurse—not to mention a patient—is evident in the story she tells years later.

It was seemingly like any other day on the floor, only it was Saturday, and so it was quiet. I was on the east side and had my usual six patients, but I wasn't very busy. I finished my morning charting and had all of my patients comfortable by noon. Only seven more hours to go! A nurse from the west side came and sat down next to me: "Jimmy's going home today," she said. "He is?" "Yeah, the ambulance is on its way." Jimmy was going home. Going home after a long battle with leukemia. The leukemia had won. He would go home with hospice to spend his last days with his family. That is what he had asked for. I was glad for him. I went to say goodbye. He was awake but only semi-aware of his surroundings. His pain medication could keep him comfortable, but not without the added effect of making him spacey. His eyes were glossy, distant. It was as if he was looking to somewhere only he could see. I was saying goodbye. He was going home so I was saying goodbye . . . He was going home to die, so I was saying goodbye.

The gift of presence is willingly given but, at times, can take an emotional toll. Consider its effect on nurses in the following example:

Early one morning I was waiting for the students in my class to arrive. They were RNs who were working toward a bachelor's degree. Most worked full time and many came directly from work. It was not unusual for students to put their heads down to rest until the entire class gathered. This morning I noticed one of the women put her head down as if to rest, picked it up almost immediately, look around, and then put it down only to lift it again. I asked her if she was all right. She looked dazed and told me, "Some nights I just don't want to be a nurse anymore." She then went on to describe what happened the night before. A young father who had choked on food was brought into the emergency room. They were unable to dislodge the obstruction and he died. This nurse had assisted with the patient and interacted with his young wife and his parents as they became aware of what had happened. The nurse said, "It was awful. There was nothing I could do. I haven't slept all night." As she told her story the rest of the class gathered, intently absorbed and supportive. It was as if a cocoon was being formed around this nurse, a cocoon composed of kindred spirits who totally identified not only with this experience but also with the truth of what it means to be a nurse. A realization of the value of her interactions that night and the comfort offered by her peers created an aura of authentic community in my classroom. I felt honored to be a part of that community.

Another nurse tells us of one specific event that stood out for her in nursing practice:

Until the past year, I was a flight nurse working on the medevac helicopter located at a major medical center. Having flown medevac trips for over 12 years there are many experiences that have touched both my heart and soul. We transported by helicopter all types of patients, from 23-week premature infants to multiple trauma patients to cardiac patients. One of the many patients that I remember was a 32-year-old man who had taken the day off from his regular job to help his brother-in-law cut trees down to clear an area to build a new home. Unfortunately, one of the trees they were cutting down fell the wrong way and landed on our patient. We were called in to transport him to the level one trauma center because he was in spinal shock and could not feel anything from the nipple line down. He could still breathe on his own, but had paralysis from the injury. We started him on high dose steroids per protocol. As we talked on the flight, I learned he had just gotten married a year ago and his wife was expecting their first child. I didn't know at the time if the steroids would return some or all sensation to his body. During the flight, I remember him asking multiple times if the paralysis would go away. I did not know what to say. All I could answer was "I don't know until we get to the E.R. and have your spine x-rayed; the doctors there will be able to tell you more." The next day I went to visit him in the E.R. and the news was not good. He had totally severed his cervical spine and the doctors had told him he would in fact be paralyzed for life. The only thing I could do was to hold his hand and cry with him. He kept on asking the "if only" questions we all do after something goes wrong. His were "if only I had not taken the day off from work, if only we had been more careful" and so on. I was heart-broken for him and stayed with him as long as I could.

Caring in nursing is not isolated to physical care, emotional care, or mental care. Nursing embodies all forms of caring, and sometimes we, as nurses, have to let our emotions show and let our patients know that we too are human. These experiences can renew an awareness of what it means to be a nurse and how nurses in a community of nurses share and understand that meaning. Being present to patients and their loved ones during times of emotional turmoil evokes emotional responses that can create distress for the nurse. Affiliation and connection to other nurses who understand and relate to this experience can ease the pain.

Here is another experience that illustrates presence and the nurturing nature of nursing:

Recovering from a year-long psychiatric hospitalization during which she delivered a beautiful baby, Jane was faced with difficult choices that would affect her and her baby. As a young mother also, I sensed and empathized with her love and concern for her baby as well as with her anxiety, which became more acute during her supervised visits with her baby. Jane was keenly aware that there were many opportunities for a good adoption placement for the baby, as there were long waiting lists for healthy infants. She also knew that she was not considered competent to take care of her baby. If she decided to keep her, the baby would be placed in foster care for years. The emotional turmoil and heart-wrenching decision to place her baby for adoption was difficult for her to live through, but Jane told me that it was made more bearable because she had me as a companion. A connection was formed as she and I, each in our own way, experienced the emotional upheavals of her dilemma. We still maintain contact. Jane is now married with two children. After a long and dedicated struggle, she has also become a competent and well-respected nurse.

From working with Jane, I came to understand that living through a profound and painful loss in the presence of another creates a human connection that provides comfort. The bond that develops may or may not persist in actuality but becomes a part of the enduring human fabric of both nurse and patient.

On another occasion, before I became a nurse, I would visit a dying relative and stay for extended periods of time. My relative had a recurrent brain tumor and was slowly slipping into unconsciousness. I watched as nurses cared for her, doing various interventions such as suctioning, IV monitoring, and grooming. I tried to do what I could to help, but it was difficult to know exactly what to do or even if it would make a difference. Yet, one nurse seemed to know that the hanging basket of flowers that she had brought in would make a difference. I watched her suction the patient, repositioning the basket from one side of the bed to the other depending on the patient's position. I sensed decreased muscle tension and lessened sounds of discomfort as this nurse attended to her. These observations comforted me. I stood in awe.

It is only recently, after many years of experience, that I am able to grasp the profundity of that nurse's activities as well as the significant impact they had on me, not only for my own nursing practice but as a model for being-in-the-world with others. The nurse used the flowers to affirm her recognition of her patient as a subjective human being, perceiving and appreciating beauty in times of imminent death. It is in these times that we are most tempted to objectify a patient as a disease or malady, rather than as a person who still exists beyond the seemingly unconscious body.

At times, nurturing and offering the gift of presence are not directed toward survival but toward accompanying others in their final journey to a dignified death.

"Can you stay a little while longer?" A feisty resident at a nursing home who had usually been oppositional and terse during rounds asked this of me one night. The uncharacteristic softness in her voice and the look in her eyes made me stop in my tracks. When I placed my hand on hers, she did not withdraw. Rather, she rotated her thumb so that it now rested on the back of my hand. We looked into each other's eyes and although there were no words spoken, the moment was intense. We both seemed to know that time was running out. I

Box 2–1 | Touch

Touch, whether physical, emotional, or spiritual, can be offered as a response to a person's call for help. Calls for help may manifest themselves in many ways—through touch, a sound, a look, a gesture. Touch can bring a feeling of closeness with another person and a sense of self-conscious affirmation of one's own identity as a nurse who has made a difference in the life or death of another.

checked her vital signs, which were unremarkable, and told her I would be back soon. I knew that she knew I would be. I was able to be with her for long periods throughout the night as she reminisced a bit about her life's journey. The usual tasks were accomplished with unaccustomed ease, but the mood did not change. As morning came I once again stood by her bedside. She squeezed my hand and we said good-bye. The next night I learned that after breakfast, she took a nap and passed away in her sleep. I smiled and felt at peace with myself.

See Box 2–1 on touch.

The Humanistic Connection

Authentic presence comprises a willingness to offer oneself as a "real" human being, an inhabitant of the Earth with others like oneself (Kleiman, 2005; Paterson & Zderad, 1976; Schutz, 1970). Authentic presence may be thought of as the way people present themselves as they truly are. Authenticity is willingness to reveal a set of attributes, values, beliefs, and concerns. These attributes have been acquired either consciously or unconsciously through life's experiences, environment, heritage, and tradition within the context of the professional yet humanistic relationships that honor both patient and nurse as unique human beings. Excluded are constructs derived solely from modern technology, politics, and socially incurred constraints that blur the essence of authentic presence.

Schein (1993) tells us that we as human beings long to participate and share in the wonders of the world with others, to present ourselves to others authentically as a statement of our reality, of our existence in the world with others. A presentation to another and a reciprocal recognition of one's self is the only way to attain self-consciousness and self-actualization. Authenticity entails each nurse using the scientific knowledge and technical skills he or she has acquired to express caring for a unique person at a particular time and place. Authenticity brings forth the art in the art-and-science equation of nursing.

Often in the world of health care the reciprocal recognition of another being like oneself is set aside as we direct our attention to a particular illness or disease and its possible causes and cures. In these cases, practitioners focus exclusively on a particular pathology and lose sight of the importance and therapeutic effect of human contact as well as the patient's entitlement to quality service and dignified treatment. Whether it is verbalized or not, each and every patient has a perception of, and an opinion about, the quality of care received or not received and the way he or she was treated by those persons administering that care.

Patients and families have come to expect a certain kind of care from nurses. This is noted in public surveys (Gallup, 2005) but more often anecdotally. For example, one student mentioned a recent experience while she was in a comedy club. The comedian asked her name and started to jibe her. When he asked her what she does, she retorted that she was studying to be a nurse. The entire audience immediately broke into applause, and the comic said that's very good and moved on to another target. The student said that that experience gave her a feeling for the awesome responsibility of being a nurse.

On another occasion, a tour guide, looking out at the Florence Nightingale Museum, recited to a nurse in the tour group the first lines of the Longfellow poem:

> Honor to those whose words or deeds
> Thus help us in our daily needs,
> And by their overflow
> Raise us from what is low!

This nurse also received applause, not as an individual person but as a person who was a nurse. This experience provides a profound statement of what it means to be a nurse in the most articulate of languages, poetry (Kleiman, 2005).

Once during an interview, I was asked what my specialty was. When I responded that my specialty is humanistic nursing, the interviewer looked surprised and asked, "Is there any other kind?"

The innuendo implicit in these occasions is that we all know that nursing is based on humanistic values, manifested in the face-to-face interactions of nurses with their patients. In today's complex and changing health-care environments, however, the notion that humanistic nurse-patient interactions are central to the nursing act is being pushed away, out of sight. The notion has become blurred by the myopic vision for the way health care should be delivered under the stresses of the day.

What is the patient's experience when this humanistic connection does not occur? Two examples of how patients perceive the way health-care professionals respond to patients' health-care concerns are given by Cameron (2002). The first is a young man who as a result of a car accident is paralyzed from the neck down. He complains that there are barriers and distance between his attending staff and himself that he experiences as being insensitive to his needs as a human being. He is angered by this state-of-affairs because he feels it deprives him of the quality of care he needs and deserves. "You're not treating me as a human being and that exercise of you professionals makes me want to die" (pp. 15–16).

The second patient complains that when he goes for his periodic hemophilia treatment as soon as the identification bracelet goes on his wrist he is treated like a number rather than as a person deserving dignified and respectful treatment. He feels that once the identification bracelet is affixed to his wrist his right to speak out on his own behalf is limited or diminished to the extent that it may affect the quality of the care he needs. Is this the way it is in our health-care systems? Do we use symbols like wrist bands and dressing gowns to signal a de-personalization and reduction of personhood of our patients? Is this a necessary result of objectifying patients in terms of a disease or malady rather than recognizing them as persons with health-related concerns who are asking for help?

On the other hand, Cameron related one occasion in which this patient experienced the human care and concern of his nurse following a night of unremitting pain that was finally responding to medication.

> He was all scrunched down in the bed, the bed clothes were in great disarray about him, and his face was covered with perspiration in response to the pain. The nurse wet a face cloth, washed his face, gently lifted his head, and turned his pillows over. She quietly left the room, put a sign on the door not to disturb him, left a message at the nursing station that he needed some sleep, and carried on with her work while constantly guarding his door like a prowling tiger cat (p. 19).

As these story illustrate, one of the fundamental truths of human centered nursing is the occasion—or, rather, the absolute necessity—of two people interacting in a shared lived experience, each recognizing the other as a living, breathing, feeling, and thinking fellow human being.

From this observation it follows that the focal point of the nurse's universe of concerns is at the face-to-face nurse/patient interaction. It is at this focal point that a nurse nurtures the patient. It is through this interaction, at this nursing occasion, that a nurse experiences the primordial truth of nursing (Henderson, 1964; Paterson & Zderad, 1976; Peplau, 1965; Kleiman, 2005).

REFERENCES

Buber, M. (1965). *The knowledge of man.* New York: Harper & Row.

Cameron, D. (2002). Ritualized experiences. In *Writing in the dark*, Ed. Van Manen, M. Western Ontario: Althouse Press.

Gallup. (2005). "Gallup's annual poll on the honesty and ethics of people in different professions." Retrieved March 10, 2006, from http://www.gallup.com

Henderson, V. (1964). The nature of nursing. *American Journal of Nursing,* 64(8): 62–67.

Kleiman, S. (2005). Discourse on humanism in nursing. *International Journal for Human Caring,* 9, 9–15.

Paterson, J. G. & Zderad, L. T. (1976). *Humanistic nursing.* New York: John Wiley & Sons.

Peplau, H. E. (1965). The heart of nursing: Interpersonal relations. *Canadian Nurse,* 61, 273–275.

Schein, E. (1993). The Academic as Artist: Personal and Professional Roots. Retrieved February 23, 2006, from www.edschein.com

Schutz, A. (1970). *On phenomenology and social relations: Selected writings.* Chicago: Chicago University of Chicago Press.

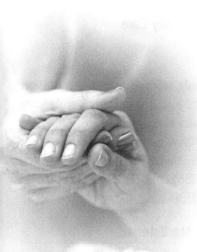

Chapter 3

Origins of Human Centered Nursing

B asic to human centered nursing is the act of one person giving aid and comfort to another. The desire to give in this manner is an inherent quality of human beings and may be observed throughout all of history. Anecdotal evidence is found in legends and stories of people reaching out to others who appeared to be in need. Responding to those who cry out in pain, sorrow, or distress is part of the empathic and sympathetic nature that is a unique characteristic of human beings.

The ancient Greeks provided some of the earliest records of the way people behaved toward each other as a constituent of the social evolution of moral and ethical behavior. They recognized the importance of human interrelationships, especially within the context of social order and community involvement and responsibility (Aristotle, 350 BC; Plato, 1945). The Greeks held that we glean an understanding of human nature by studying what people do and how they interact, especially when actions are directed toward doing good or evil to others. By others, the Greeks referred to both the actions of individuals toward one another and actions directed at or from the community within which the individuals lived.

Many of the concepts relevant to our daily lives, and especially the world of nursing, have their earliest roots in appearances of nurturing, empathy, moral responsibility, and ethics. Although not unique to nursing, human centered care is strongly held as a value of the profession (Benner & Wrubel, 1989; Green-Hernandez, 1992; Leininger, 2001; Paterson & Zderad, 1976; Watson, 1988) and easily recognized in the views of the earliest nursing professionals. For example, Florence Nightingale (1946) claimed that the essence of nursing rested on the nurse's capacity to provide humane, sensitive care to the sick within a nurturing environment that promoted health and healing. In 1948, Hildegard Peplau (1965) introduced her theory of Interpersonal Relations, which focused on the human connection between nurse and patient. She stated, "It seems to me that interpersonal relation is the core of nursing. Basically, nursing practice always involves a relationship between at least two real people, a nurse

what I think, or Jo, or you. It's really what we all think it is. So, you know, if you all saw only my view, that would be pretty dull. So to really get the fullest possible view of nursing, we should value the difference in each others' views and somehow see how they relate or how they don't relate.

JP: And I think that when we were teaching together on a master's level at Catholic U, we had a lot of seminars with students about their clinical experiences. And I think we began to really search through their clinical experiences with them. So I think we began to really focus on experience right off, when we started together—the experience of nursing. I think that's followed through all along the way. Because then later, at Ohio State, when we were asked to do something with phenomenology, with students and faculty. . . .

LZ: Right. Then, you see, we had sort of worked out our style. Because in my master's dissertation on philosophy, I wrote on Erich Fromm's theory of man, and then in my doctoral dissertation I developed a construct of empathy because I was still struggling with that notion of how is it possible for you to know the other person. How is this possible? How can you really know someone, and that's how I got into empathy. And then Jo, in her doctoral study, was trying to synthesize and compare the works of Theresa Muller and Ruth Gilbert.

JP: I was looking at their works and really using the phenomenological approach on written material. I don't know whether you people even know about the old days in psych/mental health, but they used to be almost two separate fields in Catholic U and I think other places, too. Students in one group were taught differently from how they taught the students in the other group.

LZ: It was like the public health nurses were studying mental health, and all the hospital nurses were studying psychiatric nursing, and it was like two different worlds.

JP: So, in teaching in CU, I think our emphasis got to be, how do we put it together? The underlying theory must be the same, but how do we really put programs together? We really fought to get it integrated because the National Institute of Mental Health stopped giving grants for both programs.

LZ: One group of nurses was looking at the healthy side, and the other group was more toward the pathology when we got together. As a matter of fact, when we started having public health nurses in the hospital and hospital nurses in the community, the public health nurses who were sent to the hospital would say that the patients belong in the community, and the hospital nurses who were sent to the community would say that these patients belong in the hospital.

JP: They really taught each other that people had both wellness and illness.

LZ: But I think it was experiences like this that maybe we were trying to integrate in our theory—maybe that's it—we were trying to put all these experiences together. Anyhow, when we went to Ohio State—we were both teaching in the graduate program there—some of the faculty and some of the graduate students, too, were asking us to conduct a seminar with them because they were interested in phenomenological methods of study. Some of them were trying to do studies and did their theses about doing this style rather than the positivistic, scientific, experimental approach. And I think we began to clarify it then.

JP: Around the time we were there, our article came out, which was nursology, or phenomenology or the philosophy of nursing. The students picked up that article out of nursing research and used it as a basis for their dissertations. I know one did hers on growth. She was looking into growth in nursing. Somebody else did it on a child. And others looked at other experiences.

LZ: It was like examining their own experiences with patients, and out of this they were trying to describe their styles or the major themes that were running through their work.

JP: The [woman] who did it on growth . . . was in a community mental health center. She taped her contacts with clients, and she believed that she was following Carl Rogers's philosophy. So she was looking to see whether she was pursuing his philosophy in her tapes. What she found as she listened to herself, she kept going to sleep. She all of a sudden woke up startled and realized she really wasn't interested in looking for Carl Rogers's philosophy. She was looking for her own philosophy. And as soon as she began to realize that, she stayed awake. She got very excited, but before that she was bored, and that was her dissertation on growth. Somebody else did one on a child that was mentally retarded. And the other [woman] did one on community mental health centers, something to do with how people in that socio-economic stratum communicated. So many people used it.

LZ: I remember one frightful experience with a student. In the middle of one of our sessions she grabbed and pulled off her wig.

JP: I thought she was pulling her hair out [laughter]. I think the theory sort of upset them a little bit.

LZ: And then we moved. We really wanted to get into a clinical setting, although we were supervising students in various clinical settings. As teachers, we really wanted to get back to a practice setting.[. . .] And we were consultants at a couple of VA hospitals, so one of the chief nurses said, "Why don't you come to work for the VA?" And we said it's too structured, we'll never make it. So she whipped out the map, and here was this house right in Northport on Long Island Sound, right on the sound, so that's how we got to Northport [. . .].

JP: I was reading Herman Hesse's *The Glass Bead Game.* I don't know if anybody has read that or not. But it was the idea of people getting into this game. It was a fantasy, really, and they got to be very erudite about this game. But the game began to feel like nothing. And in the end he went back to being a teacher, the man who went to the head of this game-playing. And I began to feel it at the curriculum meetings when they started drawing lines; you know, this arrow went down, and that arrow went up. I couldn't stand it anymore. And I wrote a note [to Loretta], and I said it reminds me of *The Glass Bead Game.* And I'd rather be in the clinical area.

LZ: There were a couple other things going on in academia at the time. We were teaching at Boston University when they had the riots.

JP: In the sixties.

LZ: Martin Luther King was shot. He was a graduate of Boston. They had these riots. For various reasons we moved to Ohio State, and then we were there when they had the riots at Kent State.[. . .]

JP: So it was a time of a lot of unrest, and we were feeling some need to get into clinical practice. And so that's how we got to Northport. And probably we wouldn't be hired today with the economy as it is.

LZ: At that time they were about to open a new hospital, and they had extra positions. And the chief nurse, who had a public health back-ground, was very creative and sort of said she would really like to see what could be done with doctorally prepared clinicians, and what did we want to do? And we said we would like to be like the clinical artist-in-residence. She laughed, and so I thought I better laugh. I laughed and got the job, and I never put that on my job description. That was sort of the idea.

JP: I said what I want is to get to know the people and find out what they need and what I have to contribute. That's where I was.

LZ: So that's really what we did.

JP: The administrator took a chance.

LZ: What we did was to see what was going on in the situation. I was assigned to work with staff on in-patient psychiatry and the long-term units, and Jo was working with nurses in the community and in acute care.

JP: I would say one thing for the administrator. She was very secure within herself, and she could then allow you freedom to think and "be." And she could argue back and forth with you, and she could enjoy you, and she could probably laugh at some of our theoretical ideas. But we felt very good about her, and we very much wanted her to know some of the wonderful things that were going on at Northport. And that gets into one of the first things we were asked to do when we went there, to meet with a group of evening staff. Because the evening staff—I don't know why that's true every place, but they feel neglected, like no one cares about them. So we were asked if we would meet just with a group of evening staff at 10:30 at night or something, and so Loretta and I trudged in at 10:30 at night. And they were very good groups. We really enjoyed them. Everybody would come from their units, whoever could get away, and they'd share, usually something that was current. Somebody had come having just had a death on a unit or something like that. And it would be the discussion, or they'd talk about the fact that they felt neglected, and so on. But they then brought up very beautiful experiences, and we were very inspired by them. And the administrator was always telling us about all the horrible things she heard all day. And I always remembered saying to Loretta, I wonder how they'd feel about our inviting the administrator to one of these.

LZ: They could tell her all these great things they're doing.

JP: And share some of the good things. So we said we've got to ask them first. So we did, and that was the end of that because what happened was as soon as they heard she might come, it was like, boy, we'll tell her this, and we'll tell her that. And it was like she was the authority to them, and they had to tell her everything that was wrong—like she should cure it. It was very fascinating the switch from one to the other. So we used to try to share with her some of those things.

LZ: We learned from that experience that while you could go and just talk with staff, you probably could make more progress more quickly if you had something structured or definite to focus on. Not that you lecture at them, but at least give them some ideas to relate their experience to some basic concepts or something like that. So then we were asked to meet with these nurses to work on some of the problems.

JP: I had broken my leg. As I recall, I had just broken it the day before and I was home.[. . .]

LZ: So she was home with this leg in a wet cast, and they had hired quite a few nurses with the idea of opening the general, medical, and surgical building. In the meantime, these nurses were working on psychiatric units, and they weren't prepared to work on these units, nor were they that interested in working on these units. There were some clinical problems that came up. So one day in one of the meetings, the administrator, overwhelmed with hearing three or four problems—she called me in and said, "Can't you people do something to help raise the clinical sophistication of these nurses in terms of psychiatry? Now, go home and tell Jo I'm not paying her for her legs; I'm paying her for her brain; and you two figure out a course of action on what we can do." And so I think I came home and babbled. And Jo said we've got to get this course together. We have a week to do it. So I think we were putting in everything we ever thought, and in 3 days [the administrator] said, "Where is it?"

JP: That's the way she was![. . .] And it was like panic time! What can we possibly do? And she said, "Think big."

LZ: So we did, and we planned this program that was going to take— we asked for 9 months.

JP: 300 hours!

LZ: A full day a week for 9 months or something. And at that point what was she going do with us? She said, "Try it!" So we started something new and that is inviting people, telling them this was going to be offered, would they like to come to the course?

LZ: This had never been done before at the VA. I don't know how it is in other hospital settings, but usually a list would go up, and so and so will take this in-service. And it was sort of mandated. So this was something new. Well, first we knew certain key people there who were respected by staff, and so we asked them to be in this first group of the newer people. Because we were trying to sort of bridge the gap between the experienced and the inexperienced.

JP: We had a very heterogeneous group. We'd have somebody out of an AD program; somebody out of 4-year school; somebody out of a master's program.

LZ: People told us that wasn't a good mix.

JP: But it worked out well because they really could share. I think what surprised us about that was that they could focus for a full day on clinical issues and that it didn't turn into a gripe session. But we had learned before that we had to present some kind of structured presentation and then focus on that. And that's what we did. And that was like the beginning, and we had many of those classes—I think eventually, how many years, 5 years or so, we had about 124 nurses go through. The class, naturally, was cut down. Cut down from 300 to 250 to, I think, our last four courses were 128 hours. It was still a lot. It was 16 weeks, once a week for a full day.

LZ: And so what we did was not only share—we taught in a rather simple way. But the thing that they kept saying was, "Give us examples; it's so abstract. Make it concrete." And that's what we were drawing from them: "You give us what meaning it has for you. Give us an example. Do you have an example of that?" and so on. We also, I think, exposed them to a much broader range of reading than they had been accustomed to.

JP: We also started with introductions. In those groups, which were only sometimes 10 people, it took us 3 days to get through introductions.

LZ: We always said, when you are invited to join the class, you will be expected to give a 10-minute résumé of yourself.

JP: And they would say, "Ten minutes! What can I say about myself for 10 whole minutes?"

LZ: And then it would be like an hour, an hour and a half, and they were still telling us how they got to be a nurse. But, you see, it wasn't just to get to know them, because what we were really saying is that we were trying to get them to be consciously aware of their own experiences and that we were then able to relate to them. That was the idea. So all through the class they'd say, oh, remember when you did such and such, did you experience that? And so it was a way of helping them to be aware of their experience and getting them to value it. They don't value! You know, they say well, it's only my idea or it's only my experience, but you're the only one who has the experience and if you don't share it, it's lost.

JP: And they really remembered each other's experiences. So when you asked them later how come you talked (because they had all told us they wouldn't), they'd say people listened, and people wanted to hear. And that was really what the quality of the group was, I think.

LZ: And then one assignment was trying to get them to focus on their experiences. We asked them to write. But we had a consultant who had been one of our teachers at Boston. We said we're going to have them write a paper. And she said, "Don't scare them away with a paper. Nurses don't like to write. Just ask for some paragraphs!" So we would ask each week for a paragraph. It could be just something they read— something they thought of as they were working, something they experienced in their working with patients. You know, it could have been staff or anything. And they really struggled with those, but that was really the raw data from which they found their phenomena. Because then they would do this for 5, 6, 7 weeks, and we'd say now sit down and read them, and what is the theme that's running through there? And they would find it.

JP: The fact is that they were really writing about the same thing over and over.

LZ: And those were the phenomena—their style or something basic to their view of nursing. That's how we got to these phenomena. And then eventually we would get them to develop this and study [a] phenomenon in other situations or in their reading, and they would share it, this experience, with each other.

JP: And they saw many relationships between them. That's where we, I think, thought that a scientific approach would also grow out of this phenomenological approach. There were people who told us that can't be. But what we had, what was happening within each group, would be, somebody would begin to relate their phenomena to somebody else's phenomena because they were constantly talking about how they were developing. And they all shared a paper in the end, especially the first five groups. Later, when the course got shorter, you really couldn't ask for a final clinical paper. We always continued with the paragraphs. But we could see phenomena developing in people relating one phenomenon to another. So you'd get propositions or statements; you got the phenomenon in the statement.

LZ: After several years, we had about 39 that they had described, and we were really trying to find out what to do with them. Like Jo said, you could take these phenomena and use them as constructs and develop propositions, so you could have testable theory. But our idea was that if you really followed through on the phenomenological approach, got more and more examples, described [them] more fully, then eventually you would get to the real meaning of the form of the phenomena, and then you would find the relatedness of this to others. And that's how you could develop a theory that would be descriptive, but it would still be able to develop—it would still be interrelated concepts.[. . .]

JP: [. . . .] This is what nurses said were nursing phenomena: acceptance, all-at-once, anger, authenticity, awareness, becoming, caring, change, choice, clinical, confirmation, confrontation, dedication, dialogue, dying, death, empathy, freedom, frustration, give and take, openness, patience, presence, readiness, response, responsibility, self-recognition, sustaining, touching, trust, comfort, commitment, community, laughing, crying, loneliness, nurturance, understanding, and waiting.[. . .]

LZ: Then, for a couple years, Jo and I were presenting this theory and this approach at different VA hospitals and several different universities. We were doing a lot of traveling and a lot of talking to many groups. So we would go with the idea that we would just list these phenomena and ask the nurses in the groups if they felt that any of these were important in their practice. Did they ring true for them, or were they important in their practice? And we got them to rank them. Because we were trying to get some feel for whether we were influencing nurses who hadn't taken our course. Naturally, it was an outgrowth of the kinds of things we were talking about. And the interesting thing was that one phenomenon came out first most often in every 2-day institute we did.

JP: It was awareness, which is an interesting idea that nursing would value awareness to that extent. Participants ranked the 39 phenomena. Two hundred nurses ranked 11 of these phenomena as most important in their nursing practice, and they listed them in this order: awareness, openness, empathy, caring, touching, understanding, responsibility, trust, acceptance, self-recognition, and dialogue. So that was when we ranked them. We felt that if we were giving a different kind of an institute, they would have chosen others. We also gave a pretest and post-test in those institutes. And, of course, we were testing our teaching, I think, more than we were testing what they believed in. But there was a tremendous change in the 2 days in the way they answered the questions.

LZ: But the thing that we found fascinating—when we had these groups that went 9 months, 6 months, and then I forget what the shortest one was. When we had these groups extended over many weeks, they went through a certain process. In the beginning, I think partly because of the terminology, they would say we really don't know what you're talking about. And then when they would get it, they'd say well, of course, everybody knows that that's nursing. Then we felt like we were on track with them. But then they went beyond that and said, yes, but there's more to it than that. So it was like almost, at first, not understanding at all, to a maybe, to getting to feel very comfortable with it—and then to looking deeper. When we did the 2-day workshops, the people went through the same thing in 2 days that these other groups went through. It was like the same kind of process.

JP: It was very interesting that we felt this several times, but one girl actually made us aware of it. It was in Salt Lake City, and we were giving a 2-day institute—we were talking humanistic nursing for 2 days.

We were around a long table, and this one girl sat way down at the other end, and she was very angry; she said little or nothing.[. . .] And at the end of the second day we were standing in the doorway, and most people were going out saying good-bye, thank you, whatever people say. And she walked straight up to us, and what she said was, she didn't know why she was so angry at us, but she was. She didn't really realize until she was home in the bathtub and all of a sudden she sat up straight and thought, I have all this knowledge and in the situation where I'm working, I'm not really able to apply it. She had a degree in psych, and she felt repressed or suppressed in a way. I think we had stirred up what she had initially hoped she could do.[. . .] So when we talked about some of these kinds of ideas, it really brought them all to the surface again, and she relived them. Now, she did in 2 days what we saw a lot of the people do in our long courses. We thought sometimes we were almost dealing with depression in a lot of our groups. I don't know whether that's right about all of us, but I think when we're not able to do, or be, or fulfill ourselves, we do get really down.[. . .]

LZ: There was a good ending to this story because in the second group another nurse felt the same way, so we got them together. We thought it was important that they have someone to share with or even to talk these ideas over with. And I think that's what's needed in a clinical setting. I think you learn that when you're in school you really learn from each other and from sharing with each other[. . .].

Through this dialogue the reader can get a feeling for the evolution of Paterson and Zderad's theory and the dialectic process in which they bounce ideas off each other and achieve new levels of understanding about the actualities of nursing that were significant in the development of their theory of nursing practice. It is suggested that the readers go through a similar process while reading the above dialog in order to develop their own personal theories of nursing.

The Kitchen Conference

The following is a transcription of a taped conversation with Paterson and Zderad in 2001. The dialogues are rich in interesting observations about the nature of nursing then and now, and the women discuss aspects of the historical and social contexts of nursing. The starting point of the discussion was definitions of phenomena gleaned from their previous work.

SK: I have some of the definitions of the 11 phenomena identified in your original work, but I haven't refined them. If we just go over them and you could tell me if you think that they're in keeping with the concepts that came out of your work. Originally, 39 concepts were identified. Correct?

JP: Yes.

SK: Then, when you did 2-day seminars, you brought them down to 11. You didn't consolidate the 39, but these were the 11 you said that people ranked as most important in their practice. I've struggled to write down the definitions that I've extrapolated from your work.

JP: Read them out loud. And then we might react to them.

SK: Okay. Awareness. One of the things that you said was that you were surprised that in all cases of ranking awareness was the first. For humanistic nursing practice, awareness means global apprehensions or seeing the patient as a whole, a gestalt. This requires consciousness of spontaneous perceptions: auditory, olfactory, aural, visual, tactile, kinesthetic, and visceral responses are involved, and each can convey unique meaning to man's consciousness. Awareness also includes recognition of the nurse's total response within herself to a particular patient in a particular here and now. It is a process of getting in touch with one's immediate impressions or response to reality before labeling, categorizing, or judging.

LZ: Sounds right. It's like the idea of bracketing, and you're just focusing on the responses that are there.

JP: I think that's a good definition of it. And it makes sense in terms of what we thought about it at that time.

SK: Okay! I had the association that this was really like a part of the bracketing process, too.

LZ: Yes, immediate response before labeling, categorizing, or judging.[. . .]

SK: Openness. For humanistic nursing practice, openness means an availability, readiness, and presence with receptivity to the immediate experience and its uniqueness. According to Paterson and Zderad, the nurse does not superimpose but maintains a capacity for surprise. The nurse's openness involves being open to what is and to what is not in the patient's state of being as weighed against some notion or standard of what ought to be with the intention of doing something about the difference. Openness conveys a freedom to choose, as well as a freedom from bond of habit and stereotyped responses, from routine, from the veils of the obvious. I like that.

JP: Yes, I like that, too.

SK: And that is also involved in the bracketing process?

JP: Yes, I think you have to, in a sense, bracket the biases to be that open. You have to be open to the fact that you have them.

LZ: Yes. I would agree that awareness would be bracketing your stereotypes and so on. So that you really get the impression of what's happening. And then in this openness, it would also mean that you're available, but you don't bracket everything. You could bracket what's not appropriate at that time. It's a bracketing in two different ways: bracketing to what's coming in and what's coming out.

SK: What's going out? So, in openness, you're bracketing your responses?

LZ: You're being open to what is and what is not.

JP: I think you have to be open to your responses. And if they were inappropriate, you wouldn't act on them.

LZ: You're saying, freedom to choose, as well as a freedom from the bonds of habit and stereotyped response. In other words, you don't just give a usual response. Or you hold your stereotypes while you respond to what's here.

SK: From what you just said, it's like the intellectual piece of it is being held in abeyance, but you're allowing your intuitive to be open. You grasp.

JP: I think you're always letting your intuitive be open. What you do with it is another thing.

LZ: That's what I was trying to say. In other words, you're free from the bonds of habits, stereotyped response, routine veils of the obvious. You don't just fit things in.

JP: I wonder, Loretta, if you could use an example like the one you gave of going into the ladies' room. And your idea in this example was that you should be respectful and not undo the attendant's work.

LZ: Not mess up her clean floors and polished basins.

JP: But you were open to what she said, which was completely the opposite of how you had perceived the situation.

LZ: So I must have said it in a way that didn't stifle her. Even if it was unusual for anyone to say this or to consider her, she could tell me, "Really if you don't mess it up, if you don't do it, I don't have a job." So it was like an openness both ways.

SK: To who she is.

LZ: That's right.

JP: Yes, and you were very accepting of her as to who she was.

LZ: And what she was doing.

SK: So it entails acceptance.

JP: I think so. Acceptance of when the person is open with you, you don't write them off. You really accepted her.

SK: Okay. So, basically, what you were talking about with openness is this sense of acceptance with regard to [people] as they are.[. . .] I also found it in your paper on empathy, Loretta.[. . .]

JP: Loretta did a whole dissertation on empathy.

SK: This is one that you didn't define in the back of the book.

LZ: [. . .] See, empathy also really fits that other example of the woman in the washroom. Initially I was imagining myself in that situation, not oneness with the other by sharing his being in a situation resulting in knowledge of his perspective. I, however, got her perspective because . . . .

JP: You were open.

LZ: I was open.

JP: That's why they all flow into together.

LZ: They do. They're all related—awareness, acceptance, and openness.

SK: But you couldn't have been empathic if you weren't open.

JP: That's right.

SK: Right? And you couldn't have been open if you weren't aware.

JP: Aware. Right. So that's what I mean. I have a hard time separating them.

SK: That's the all-at-once.

LZ and **JP:** Yes . . . right.

SK: You're up and down, back and forth, all at once. Right?

JP: That's how I got that.

In the following segment, the discussion turned to nursing today as compared to when Paterson and Zderad did their original work.

SK: Now, let's look at what's happening now. Based on all the changes within the world—the information explosion, technology, etc.—are nurses still experiencing those things that you identified in your work, or are they experiencing other things?

JP: Well, I had a very hard time when both Loretta and our friend Sue were in the hospital because nurses would come in the morning and say, "I'm Ms. So-and-So, and I'm your nurse for today," and I never saw them again. And an administrator said to me, "Well, they are supervising the other people, you know, the 15 people that come in all day long, all these different people."[. . .]

LZ: The problem was, when she says "I'm your nurse today," we think of how we were a nurse.[. . .] It's very different now.[. . .]

JP: I don't know that she, my idea is then, she's really not your . . .

LZ: . . . not my nurse.

JP: No. She's supervising the people who are caring for you.

LZ: Even if she said that, I would have different expectations. But if she comes and says "I'm your nurse today," I would expect to see her. But if she came in and said, "Well, I'm in charge of your care, but other people will be doing it, and I'll be in touch with them, but you could call me if you need me." You know, something like that. But see, I don't know what people expect. I don't know if that's because I expect that because that's the kind of nursing I did. Maybe an ordinary person doesn't expect that.[. . .]

JP: Yes. Then the other part of that, "I'm your nurse for today, I'm Miss So-and-So," reminds me of, "I'm Evelyn, and I'm your server." And I get very mixed up with some of this stuff because that is such a rote kind of thing to say. . . .

LZ: [. . .] I guess it's depersonalizing. . . .

JP: It's very depersonalizing just to go to everybody and say, "I'm your nurse for today."

SK: Yet we talk about the fact that [a nurse] is the one that is providing the individualized treatment. I mean, that's what nursing is trying to lay a claim to. Are we falling short of that?

JP: Well, there are these people up here who think nursing is this, and then there's these working bees down here and never the twain shall meet. It is a completely different idea.

LZ: That's what I'm saying. Is it that we are just so tied into that old idea of what a nurse does, or is it that when we don't see it, we think it's bad?

SK: But what you're saying also is, is there this intersubjective transactional relationship?

LZ: It's not there. It's not there. It's not an openness because she didn't connect. She gave a stereotype response and routine greeting.

JP: She doesn't see herself in the role of really relating to you.

LZ: No.

SK: And I go back to—in nursing we keep talking about the holistic. The concern being, with all the technology and all of these levels of supervising in an effort to maintain competencies, that piece of it may have almost vanished, and now is nursing going to be defined in some other way?

JP: Is she open to the people under her? Is she using these same responses? Maybe Sue's experience illustrates some of this. She had spinal anesthesia, an epidural. And they left it in after the surgery. Now they came in to look at specific machines all day long.

LZ: Different ones. . . .

JP: Different ones I mean—she had intravenous going, and I don't know what all else.

LZ: Some nurses came in to look at that, and some came in to look at another. . . .

JP: She had a catheter, all kinds of stuff. But she got to the point of pain before they realized her epidural was leaking. So nobody really checked her. It was dripping. But it was dripping into the bed.

LZ: And it wasn't until she really said she's had a lot of pain that they checked.[. . .]

SK: I wonder what the supervising nurse or the nurse that was in charge of her care experienced in relationship to that piece of her nursing care, because she's identifying you as her patient?

JP: The evening nurse fixed it, and Sue thought she was great.

LZ: But did she ever see her again?

JP: I don't know. Well, I think she did because I think evenings and nights are different.

LZ: Yes. That's another thing.

JP: That's another whole routine.

LZ: They don't have all those levels of people coming in.

JP: Yes, there aren't 15 different people coming in.

SK: And that was experienced from the patient's point of view, from Sue's point of view, as a more positive experience?

JP: Right. And the interesting part of that is, I was talking to this friend of mine, and what she said was that some nurse told her she wanted to work nights, because you didn't have to work on nights. And she didn't have to put up with all the difficulties of the day shift. So there it is—it's very confusing because you could probably have patient contact at night if you wanted it, but you wouldn't have to deal with all the different departments in the hospital, the doctors and all the rest of them—I don't know what the answer is to all this.

SK: I don't know if the experience of nursing today . . .

JP: . . . is the same at all.[. . .]

SK: I mean, whether it's a sense of responsibility gone awry or something else, I don't know. You know your work was really pre–managed care. Managed care really hadn't taken a hold of the world. Even in the other tape you talk about the fact that times were changing as you moved into your new positions at the VA. The change was based on the fact that the system just couldn't afford, at that point in time, to support nurses in the clinical field doing theoretical work. It was a much more practical-driven time. . . .

SK: Now, with managed care, with all the technology. . . .

LZ: Yes, actually—we were doing a talk a while ago, and we were talking about empathy and this kind of care, and one of the nurses said, "Where are you going to get an administrator to pay for that?" I think that's where we are now. And yet maybe they're doing it but in a different way. I don't know.

LZ: Well, this young master's student who just called from Ohio—he's studying to be a nurse practitioner, and he wants to eventually go into private practice. Because this is what he wants to do, work with patients. So maybe this is only possible in that kind of a situation, not in the hospital situation.

JP: It's interesting because I remember when I was in training . . . we looked down our noses at private duty nurses. We thought that they really didn't want to work.[. . .] And technically, they're the ones who were giving the best people care.

LZ: They were the real nurses.

JP: Yes. They wanted to be involved with the patient.

LZ: We were doing the functional.

JP: Yes, you almost felt like you just weren't really "with it." On the other hand, you didn't really want to be an administrator.

JP: But that's what was valued. Those are the ones that got the better salaries, etc. So we didn't really value the caregivers.

LZ: It's very mixed up.

SK: Right. And now the idea is clinical nurse specialists are becoming nurse practitioners who have collaborative agreement with physicians.

JP: I think and hope there would probably be safeguards for the nurse practitioner to have autonomy. And I don't know why we would necessarily be controlled by that agreement, but I would like the cooperation that it would entail. I don't know why we're so against working with other people. I mean, that seems okay with me as long as it isn't an authoritarian-slave relationship.

SK: The role of the nurse practitioner will evolve, but physicians expect the nurse practitioner to help them understand what the role is. And since nurses have never functioned as nurse practitioners before, it may be very difficult for them to define it.

JP: That's the way I experienced public health. When you would call a physician when you were in the community and ask him for orders for something or tell him what the situation was, first off many of them would say no. They don't want a nurse going in there. That was the initial response. The second response was when the doctor came upon a patient who really needed patient care—needed a lot of help, then he'd call you. Once he experienced what you were doing in the situation, he became your friend, and you worked together, and you shared.

LZ: You respected each other.

JP: It was a process that went on. But it's not too different than what you're saying today, really. I think the way that nurse practitioner thing was set up was as an extension of the doctor rather than a collaborative relationship between two professionals.

SK: It was supposed to let [nurses] get into the arena. There was so much resistance on the part of the physician because it was seen as a threat, reducing the number of physicians that would be necessary.

JP: [. . .] That was exactly how a public health nurse was viewed. She went into the home and gave all the health education, she treated the patient, etc. They saw us as taking over their jobs. But once they really needed a nurse in there and she really did work well with them, it was a whole different story. You'd get call after call then from the same guy.

LZ: And a lot of this is cultural, you know, bound by our system. A nurse who studied nursing in Britain and then came over here found the kind of relationships we had with doctors so hard because in England it was different. She thought it was the way our schools started. Florence Nightingale set up schools of nursing, and the nurse was in charge of the unit. That was her domain, and the physician came into her domain, whereas here, nurses were considered part of the hospital, and the doctors controlled the hospitals and were in charge of the schools and did a lot of the teaching. And so we started out in this . . .

JP: . . . hierarchical. . .

LZ: . . . different kind of subservient role to the doctor, whereas they didn't have that.

JP: No, that nurse matron of the school was the boss.

SK: That's interesting because I did pick up some of that in the historical review.

LZ: If that was her unit, her domain, she was in charge. And the doctor had to fit in.

JP: You can read about it in any book.

SK: And in today's arena, though, you have not only the doctor . . .

LZ: . . . the administrator . . .

SK: . . . you have the managed care company.

LZ: Okay. So that's another whole level.

SK: That's another dictator who comes in and influences what the nurse does. Today we have courses in the hospitals on managed care so that the nurses understand the financial aspects of what's going on. I don't remember that being mentioned in my initial training, but that was never an emphasis during that time.

LZ: So you might not even find these phenomena identified in our work at all today.

SK: I might not. I may find some and not others, or I may find something entirely different.

LZ: Yes.

JP: Our work was related to everybody in nursing.[. . .] As far as what I taught them, I'd say most of it came out of the community rather than out of my psych experience in a hospital, which was very limited.

SK: I personally know from my experience, I use it in all areas.[. . .] I may use it when I'm being an administrator.

JP: So did I as a teacher educator.

SK: Right, any meeting that I'm at, I use the principles.

LZ: She's saying it's not psych.

JP: It's not.

SK: It's nursing.

JP: Nursing, right. I feel that very strongly. You need to say that. And I think Teresa Muller would have said that, and she was not a psych nurse. That's why she wrote it's for all of nursing.[. . .]

SK: No, and I can point that out that the people that were involved in your original workshops were not all from Psych. I think some of the phenomena identified might be more related to other types of nursing than psych nursing—like the touching, for example. Touching in psych does happen, but it's not the same type.

JP: It's not taking care of a colostomy.

SK: It's not the same intrusion.

JP: Or it's not a mastectomy. It's a whole other area. And all of these apply to it.

SK: And yet, I think that touching is an important aspect in all of nursing.

JP: Touching isn't always just physical, either.

SK: See, now that's why I'm having such a hard time with the definition of touching. [. . .] What do we mean by touching? It's not always just physical touching. It's also. . . .

JP: Psychological touching or whatever—I don't know—or a whole human response. Because I think of that colostomy patient I took care of. You could say I was touching her colostomy. But you could also say that I touched her when I didn't use the word colostomy when she couldn't come up with it. But she went through a whole bunch of sounds before she got to colostomy. That's when it touched her. How did I know? She said after, "This is the first time I've eaten a full meal since I had the surgery. This is the first time." I don't know what I did, but . . . she was the one who finally said it. . . . So I touched her in a way. And I don't know how to say it, but I think that's touching a person even if I didn't put a hand on her. That's what I mean. That's the broad definition of touching.

LZ: I think of when something happens and people say, "Oh, I'm touched." And they don't mean physically touched. It's something you did or said or . . .

JP: . . . had meaning for them, real meaning.

LZ: So that's when touching . . .

SK: . . . has almost a visceral meaning then.

LZ and **JP:** Yes, right.

SK: I mean because it's more than conscious, it's almost like a . . .

JP: . . . whole body reaction, a visceral reaction to the person. That's what I would mean by touching. You think you can find a definition for all of that?

LZ: I'm trying to think of examples. You know, when I felt touched but not physically touched . . . It's being moved, isn't it?[. . .] or like really being understood.

JP: Well, it gets right back to empathy again. That person really experiences your empathy—your openness or whatever.

SK: But is empathy more intellectual and touching more primitive?

JP: More primitive?

SK: [. . .] I was listening to the radio the other day, and some song came on about Indians, about they're being killed off and their culture being killed, and I could feel, I was touched. I had no intellectual under-standing of what happened.

LZ: Yes. I can remember at that workshop in the Berkshires that we had from Boston University. It was on the arts in nursing, the value of the arts in nursing. And at one session I went to there was a young pianist and he was playing. It started out with something like "Moon Over Miami" or something like that kind of song. Then, all of a sudden, it changed into something almost mean. It was like his response was when people marched in the South, during the civil rights movement, and soldiers took over. I remember I was so shocked I couldn't get over it for a couple of hours.

SK: You were touched.

JP: The music got to you.[. . .] Being touched is to have your emotions open.

LZ: Yes, I think so. And, like they say, music is the universal language, you know. I don't think of myself as particularly musical or understand-ing music, but it was an understanding, it was responding. So that's what touch is, responding emotions and even more.[. . .] You don't have to put it into words. So you don't have to intellectualize or label it. A touch could be touched in all kinds of ways. You could be hurt or you could get a tremendous insight because you'd be aware of it.

SK: But it does include the physical also?

JP: Oh yes.[. . .]

SK: Now the other one is caring. Now, you know, some of the theo-rists today have identified caring as the hallmark of nursing.

LZ: You mean the doctor is curing?

SK: Right, but I'm not exactly sure, and I'm not exactly clear, how the nurses in your data identified caring.

LZ: Isn't it spelled out anywhere?

JP: I don't even remember. Did we do much with caring in the book?

SK: No, not in the book.

LZ: Not in the original book. I like the introduction to that—the foreword to the original book. This was by Lilyan Weymouth and she said, "Nursing even sings very softly because our ears are attuned to a different drummer (Paterson & Zderad, 1976, p. vii)." In other words, just because it's different, don't reject it.

JP: Yes.

SK: Caring was one of the top 11 named by the nurses in your workshops.

LZ: We got off on that by touching. Touching and caring . . .

SK: Caring, I could be wrong, but I get the sense of the whole person—helping people be all that they can be in the situation that they are in is a form of caring.

JP: Right, but that also was my definition of comfort.

SK: Okay. And that's what I keep gravitating toward. And as you can tell by the way I gave the definition, that's what I think caring is.

LZ: This is hard.

SK: It wasn't put into that word, but that's what all of this is, or is caring the actual *doing* part of what the nurse does? It's almost as though that it's some kind of action or activity or something that's done that's other-directed—focused on another.

JP: I remember people thinking comfort was trivial. Well, if care isn't what you're talking about, I mean, you wouldn't go through all these steps that I defined in my dissertation, the 12 nurse behaviors that I view as comfort, you wouldn't go through all those unless you cared. As I look at them I think, well, who the heck would do this if they didn't care?

SK: So that's all part of caring, it's an action, it's manifest. But the caring can be nonaction, right, like you can care. A nurse can care even if she can't do anything about it. She can care if you have a miscarriage, but then does she do anything?

LZ: I see what you're saying. Are we talking about physical caring here, nursing care, or are we talking about emotional care?

SK: I think it's the same process we just went through with touching. You know what I'm saying?

JP: Yes. Right. That's interesting because you could make that kind of a point.

SK: And those were the two that I couldn't really grasp. But I think it's that same kind of basic issue. Caring, like touching, can be doing it or an emotional response, and you don't necessarily have to observe it.

LZ: You could also do something in a way that the person thinks you don't care.

JP: Again, you get into the well-being, which signifies a particular mode of being and a particular kind of cognitive knowledge with all his human capacity—the clinician relates with his clinical world consciously, deliberately. See, to me, it's caring, yes.

LZ: And I think you just said, Jo, it's being clinical or consciously and deliberately an I-thou and an I-it. But wait. What you just said is a state of being as well as . . .

JP: . . . Yes, a state of being and a particular kind of cognitive knowledge and I think that's true. But that . . .

LZ: It's being and doing, and we're struggling with how to define the being part. And you could do the doing part of it without having, for example, a burned-out nurse or someone who's gotten quite cynical. They could still go through the routines—the nurse-caring routines.[. . .] I think caring has two dimensions—the actual doing of something and the underlying—would it be attitude? It's one of those things that you almost can define more easily when it's not there.

SK: You can define it through its absence.[. . .] I think about some of the nurses that I work with and when they even talk about doing things like calling up SSI and making an appointment for somebody because the benefits are running out, it's a very mechanical thing. But you experience the caring on the part of the person that's doing it.

JP: Yes.

LZ: This . . . 40-year-old nurse in a master's program . . . said he was trying to give an example. He works in the emergency room. And he went by a door or a cubicle or something. Anyhow, this patient's IV was running right. This is what he told me: "She wasn't my patient, but I went in and I adjusted the IV and I don't know what else. And she said, 'Oh, I wish you were my nurse. I'd like to have a nurse like you.'" And he said, you know, the idea was I cared enough to do this. So it was a sense of responsibility that would move you to do something if you cared. Or if you couldn't do anything, at least express something.

JP: . . . This definition seems to me to be important—presence. Are you working at all with presence?

SK: It wasn't listed at all as one of the 11.

JP: But I was wondering if you could get it in some way.

SK: I'm going to put it in the concepts.

JP: Okay. You have this? "A mode of being available or open in a situation with what I like was a gift of the self."

LZ: Yes.

JP: Because I was thinking that's sort of what caring is about. It can only be given freely, invoked or evoked.

LZ: Get that down. Don't lose that thought.

JP: It's under the definition of presence.

LZ: I think that given freely . . .

JP: Yes.

LZ: . . . invoked, they call it forth.

JP: Yes, right.

LZ: But somebody else could be in that situation and wouldn't feel. . . .

JP: It reminded me of the example you just gave of the graduate nurse. He did it of his own free will. In other words. . .

LZ: He saw the need.

JP: Right. So he was open to this person's need, and he invoked or evoked that.

LZ: It's like that call-and-response thing.

JP: Yes, call-and-response. Yes.

LZ: They are all interrelated.

JP: They are. I don't know how you separate them out.

SK: I did a review of the literature. I noticed that in the things that came back, a lot of where you're quoted are in articles related to presence.

JP: Presence. Yes. Presence has really come into being.

SK: What you're saying really is, caring is an expression of presence in being with the patient.

JP: Yes.

LZ: I think that it's invoked or evoked and. . .

JP: . . . somehow or other the patient calls it forth from you.

LZ: Once Jo and I and my aunt were visiting a cousin who was blind. And he said something to my brother about me. He said, "She's a very caring person. I can see that. You wonder how I see it, don't you?" And he was blind. So what did he really see? Because he could maybe make out an image if somebody was there. But how would he see this? It must be something that is communicated without seeing. And I wasn't really feeling like I was caring for him. I probably was responding to some other things that he was saying or going through.

JP: So there's a responsiveness involved in it.

LZ: It's a response that's invoked or evoked.

JP: And he received it.

LZ: Yes, I wonder, does it have to be received?

JP: It isn't always, no.

LZ: It isn't always interpreted as caring.

JP: No, it isn't.

LZ: So, is it still caring?

JP: Sure.

LZ: Maybe more so.

JP: Maybe that is the way children mature, that eventually they begin to experience your caring. Take the idea of the adult who has never been cared for. What are they like? Or they could have been cared for and not been able to receive it.

SK: So what you're saying is that people express caring in different ways and people receive the sense of caring in different ways. But is there something unique to caring in nursing? Because it does need to be.

LZ: It is purposeful.

JP: I think caring in nursing is sort of specific in terms of you're there for a purpose. I agree with that.

SK: But it's still basically the idea that you're expressing caring in a particular way that the patient may not perceive as caring, but . . . still a response that's evoked in you, the nurse, based on all your knowledge, experience, etc.

JP: Like the man who swore at me at 5 o'clock on a cold night when the crows were all making noise, and the patient was sitting on the steps outside the gym at Northport. And I was walking over to Loretta's office. And it was fall, and it was cold. I was new in Northport, and this little old patient was sitting curled up on a cement step outside the gym. And he looked so miserable. And I said hello, and he said, "Get out of here; you dirty son-of-a-bitch!" [laughter] I could've cried. But I think I cared about him, and I empathized with him. I thought he looked miserable. Maybe he was delighted to be away from all the patients and out on the cement steps. Who knows?

SK: But that was an expression of your caring.

JP: Yes, right. Now, whether it was received or not. . . . And yet you don't know that it wasn't.

SK: Yes.

JP: You don't really know.

This informal dialogue gives us a rich historical context for Paterson and Zderad's work and at the same time explores and compares that context with contemporary nursing issues. The dialogue introduces and discusses many of the nursing phenomena identified in their original work. Together, these dialogues provide readers with a rich background as they embark on a voyage to human centered nursing. See Box 3–2, definitions of the 11 phenomena from Paterson and Zderad's original work.

Box 3–2 | Definitions of the 11 Phenomena From Paterson and Zderad's Original Work*

1. Awareness. Awareness for humanistic nursing practice means global apprehension of the patient and the patient in his environment. Awareness entails the nurse "getting in touch with her immediate impression or response to reality before labeling, categorizing, or judging it."
2. Openness. Openness means a receptivity to the patient as he presents. It involves "making room" within oneself to allow the other to come in.
3. Empathy. Empathy in humanistic nursing is conceived of as entering into the world of the person being nursed to understand his experience of the world. It is through empathy that we come to know the other as a whole person rather than as an object.
4. Caring. Caring is perceived as the response to the call from the patient for help. It is a nurturing response on the part of the nurse directed toward helping with being and becoming.
5. Touching. Touching in humanistic nursing practice means invoking or evoking a sense of connectedness and emotional response from the patient and/or the nurse. It may be initiated by tactile or emotional stimuli.

continued

Box 3–2 | Definitions of the 11 Phenomena from Paterson and Zderad's Original Work*—cont'd

6. Understanding. Understanding in humanistic nursing practice is the integration of intuition and intellectual analysis. It is a process that allows for the assimilation of new ideas in relationship to previous knowledge and experience.

7. Responsibility. Responsibility in humanistic nursing practice means the recognition by the nurse that the nurse-patient relationship is encumbered with professional obligations.

8. Trust. In the nurse-patient relationship, trust refers to the patient's "instinctive unquestioning belief in and reliance upon" the nurse in health-wellness situations.

9. Acceptance. Acceptance in humanistic nursing practice means the nurse's willingness to receive and allow the self and the other to exist uniquely in the world. Acceptance recognizes a person's right to decide responsibly for oneself.

10. Self-recognition. Self-recognition in humanistic nursing practice means the acknowledgement of the nurse that she is first a human being. She brings all of her past experiences, all of her current being, and all of her hopes, dreams, and fears of the future that are experienced in her own space/time dimension into the nurse-patient relationship.

11. Dialogue. Dialogue is viewed as a communication in terms of call and response related to health-illness conditions. Dialogue involves every mode of human communication: verbal, tactile, artistic creations. Nursing dialogue is characterized by the unique feature of occurring through nursing acts, simplest to most dramatic.

*These definitions have been reviewed and approved by Paterson and Zderad.

REFERENCES

Benner, P. & Wrubel, J. (1989). *The primacy of caring.* New York: Addison Wesley.

Green-Hernandez, C. (1992). Being there and caring: a philosophical analysis and theoretical model of professional nurse caring in rural environments. In *Rural health nursing: stories of creativity, commitment, and connectedness,* edited by P. Winstead-Fry, et al. New York: National League for Nursing. (pp 31-53)

Henderson, V. (1964). The Nature of Nursing. *American Journal of Nursing,* 64(8): 62–67.

Hott, L. & Garey, D. (1988). Sentimental women need not apply: A history of the American nurse (VHS). Los Angeles: Florentine Films.

Leininger, M. (2001). A mini journey into transcultural nursing with its founder. *Nebraska Nurse,* 34(2), 16–17.

Nightingale, F. (1946). *Notes on nursing: What it is and what it is not.* Philadelphia: J.P. Lippincott.

Paterson, J. G. & Zderad, L. T. (1976). *Humanistic nursing.* New York: John Wiley & Sons

Peplau, H. E. (1965). The heart of nursing. Interpersonal relations. *Canadian Nurse,* 61, 273–275.

Plato. (1945). *The Republic,* trans. Francis MacDonald Comford. New York: Oxford University Press.

Watson, J. (1988). *Nursing: Human science and human care.* New York: National League for Nursing.

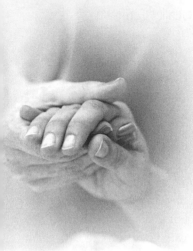

Chapter 4

Conceptual Framework of Human Centered Nursing

A conceptual framework may be thought of as a composition of interrelated ideas or concepts that serves to contextualize a particular phenomenon or event. Defining a conceptual framework in the construction of any scholarly work in nursing enhances opportunities for others to understand the message of the work as it is being related by the author. When the constituents of a conceptual framework are bound together by a set of interrelationships that present an image to the mind as a whole, rather than a set of distinct elements, we may refer to it as a structure or gestalt.

Concept Development and Analysis of Human Centered Nursing

What are concepts? A concept is an idea or a set of terms or meanings that a writer defines and assigns a name. Concepts are often called the building blocks of theory. The concept may be one that has been used previously in literature; it may represent a new, original idea; or it may be one that has been used previously but is now nuanced for a particular context. Concepts have historical, cultural, political, and socially grounded meanings in specific domains of relevance. They are historical in the sense that they derive from intellectual traditions in which their meanings have become customary. They have become customary, in part, because their meanings are embedded in each field of study (Alford, 1998, 33).

The practical purpose of concept definition is to help the reader understand what a writer means by the use of certain terms. Concept elaboration gives insight into the perspectives that color the explanations of the content and clarify further what is meant when using certain terms. Take, for example, the concept of "caring." It is necessary to define the concept in terms of 'caring for' as a mechanical process, 'caring about' as an attitude, caring demeanor, caring as a state of being, and so forth. In this way, the reader can appreciate the framework within which caring is being discussed. It is important to point out that for students embarking on a scholarly paper, research project, thesis, or dissertation, specifying a conceptual framework is a vital aspect of their presentation (Schutz, 1970, 278–279).

Theory, Concepts, Data

Concepts, once named and defined, are couched in some definite context. Every phenomenon, as is the case of human centered nursing, has both theoretical and empirical significance. The concepts facilitate movement in a back-and-forth dialectic process between reflection about the larger implications of the theoretical and philosophical domains of relevance and the concrete, evidence or data (Alford, 1998, 28–29).

For example, the theory might explain the extent to which patients' perception of the quality of interactions with their nurses varies based upon attention to and respect for patients' cultural affinities. At the highest level of abstraction, the theoretical or philosophical domains of human centered nursing include Humanism, Existentialism, and Phenomenology.

- The tenets of Humanism illuminate the value of the unique individual and the responsibility that human beings have toward each other. People who have chosen to become nurses fulfill that responsibility through their professional interactions with patients. Humanism is integrated with an existential understanding of the patient's and nurse's lived-in-world and the meanings that they ascribe to their experiences.

- Existentialism postulates that human beings are the entities that "stand-out" among all other entities in the world and who possess the unique ability to "wonder," to make choices and to take responsibility for those choices. Wonderment is the activity through which one comes to a personal perception, or understanding of the way that individuals relate to other individuals and to the social orders in which they find themselves.

- Phenomenology as a philosophy is concerned with the lived experience of human beings and the meaning that those lived experiences hold. First, phenomenology focuses on aspects of experiences (phenomena), whether real or imagined, that come into consciousness. Second, it is concerned with illuminating the fundamental truths of existence concealed in and by those phenomena. Third, it offers possibilities for discovering the fundamental nature of the nursing experience as it is relevant to each individual nurse.

Nursing is a phenomenon that entails the human-to-human connection with another, one of whom (nurse) has made the commitment to be of service to the other (patient). The phenomenon of nursing entails both a process and the meanings embedded in the experience of the connection between the nurse and patient. Three concepts make up the conceptual framework of human centered nursing: pathic touch, concern, and practical wisdom.

Pathic Touch

Nurses care for individuals, who live in a body that exists in a world of others and objects. From an existential point of view, individuals experience themselves as separate from others and, at times, alienated and alone. Health-related concerns often exaggerate this sense of loneliness and separation, creating stress and interfering with the ability to heal and cope.

The pathic touch is the fundamental means to overcome separation or barriers between nurse and patient. The pathic touch facilitates a connection between one person and another; opening a dialogue within which the patient is moved toward a better state-of-being-in-the-world. Keep in mind that the message of the pathic touch may be conveyed as a physical, emotional, or even spiritual phenomenon in the form of bodily contact, verbal utterance, silence, or even a gesture or facial expression. The pathic touch engenders a particular kind of relationship between nurse and patient that illuminates the patient's identity as a unique individual rather than an object of some disease or illness.

For example, instead of the 17-year-old male above-the-knee amputee in room 23, the patient is John, the 17-year-old varsity high school football player who is just waking up from surgery for an above-the-knee amputation of his right leg as a result of an automobile accident in which he was driving and his best friend died. This awareness of and approach to the person as an individual focuses on the pathic touch as an entry point into a human centered caring relationship. Moving from the pathic touch as an entry point to the human centered relationship helps the nurse grasp the situation from the patient's points of view. It is one of the ways nurses come to know patients' perceptions of their experiences, as well as a way nurses come to know themselves as nurses. Van Manen (1999) identifies this as the pathic or lived dimensions of the other's experiences, characterized by a reciprocal "feeling" received by nurses as they touch their patients (physically, emotionally, or subjectively). In having a feeling for someone, there is always present at the same time a self-feeling, and in this self-feeling is a mode of becoming revealed to oneself.

The pathic touch anticipates the fundamental precondition of human existence as each individual recognizes the other as a like being and provides the "yes" to the patient, the "Yes, I recognize you as a unique human being, and I want to help you. It is safe to connect with me; let me go through this situation with you." An example of an experiential epiphany about pathic touch is given here by a nursing student:

> The young couple came in with their 4-month-old baby boy. He was born with Down's syndrome. My instructor needed to explain to them the outcome of the tests. They were here for counseling and also for the baby's general check-up. The young parents looked anxious. Their baby sensed it and was getting uneasy. This was my first encounter with a baby with this syndrome. Of course, I was curious and eager to apply my knowledge and perform all the routine tests to evaluate and grade his deficiency and normal development.
>
> Yet, the mother's eyes were desperately asking for momentary relief. They were speaking from her heart. In that moment I read from a human-to-human approach: "Please, he is my first son, not a guinea pig." I empathically looked at her. I could see her pain, her anger, her frustration. I extended my arms toward her and offered to hold her son while she and her husband spoke with the doctor.
>
> I held that baby like my own. I spoke to that child with tender love. He and I became "buddies" right away. We had connected. I wasn't performing any physical exam. I was healing an unseen pain. I was not rejecting or prejudicing this child. I was there just to hold him and alleviate the anxiety of a whole family. Or maybe I was just treating my own anxiety. That day I felt beautiful. I had made contact. I had healed. I had not cured.

Concern

Concern is the awareness of human engagement with phenomena that present against people in the conduct of their daily activities. Phenomena include inanimate things, events, or people—potential, actual, real or imagined—that come into consciousness, through the senses, mystically, historically, or by way of faith. In general, a phenomenon may be thought of as something that can be spoken or thought about as it has been objectified in consciousness, like the experience of healing described above, or giving birth. A chair, table, or other solid object might also be examples of objects of consciousness.

"World" in human centered nursing is not the planet Earth, the universe, or some other abstract spatial or temporal reference point. Rather, it is a composition of everyday concerns and interests of an individual, such as the "world" of the mother or the "world" of the nurse. Being "in" such a world necessitates a practical engagement with the meaningful concerns and interests of that world. For example, the person Anna as mother thrives and participates in a different world from the same Anna as nurse. The difference is related to her distinct concerns and goals (nurturing children versus attending to patients) and the possibilities and requirements they generate. Each of her worlds consists of a dynamic set of relationships, which lend significance to the phenomena that Anna encounters. Patients, families, and others also thrive within some loosely bounded lived-in-worlds structured as dynamic sets of relationships and concerns that lend significance to the activities in which they participate, including health related activities.

In human centered nursing, nurses strive to relate to their patients and families in these lived-in-worlds, engaging in a process of, metaphorically speaking, going through life together. Relating in this way provides insight into patients' perception of their health related concerns and the treatments that they will or will not accept, as well as their perceptions of those persons giving the treatments.

Ways of being-in-the-world that have relevance for nursing and have concern as their mode of being-in-the-world are characterized as taking-care, concern-for-self, and concern-for-others (Heidegger, 1927).

Taking-Care (Concerns About Things)

Of necessity, nurses deal with errands and other matters on a day-to-day basis, such as maintaining supplies and equipment, attending staff meetings, performing evaluations, and parking their cars. Some frequently occurring examples related by nurses include: getting a meal for a patient who was brought the wrong food, searching around for a working stethoscope, and rebooting a down computer terminal. These tasks function as part of "taking care."

Concern-for-Self

Generally, in everyday activities, a person is presented with challenges from phenomena that are manifested as usual or unusual, known or unknown, manageable or unmanageable, and expected or unexpected. When confronted with the world and other people, the individual feels anxiety and dread, particularly with respect to uncertainties about what will or will not happen next.

In particular, nurses experience apprehension (concern) about possible situations that may threaten their safety; reflect on their competence, self-image, or endurance; or wonder about particular treatment or intervention situations. For example, in psychiatric nursing, a nurse may be apprehensive when a patient is psychotic and there is a loss of a shared sense of reality and ordinary symbols take on idiosyncratic meaning.

Concern-for-Others

This is the kind of concern necessarily found in nursing. It is guided by consideration and forbearance and is characterized by competently intervening for patients, standing in for them, or serving as advocate for them. This kind of concern pertains essentially to an authentic valuing that emphasizes the existence of the other as a unique person, not the what (disease or condition) with which a person is occupied. Concern-for-others proves to be a state of being-in-the-world that entails possibilities for being in and relating to the world of others and likewise with an authenticity in being oneself (Heidegger, 1927).

The following personal event characterizes both concern-for-self and concern-for-others and exemplifies the interrelated nature of the concepts of human centered nursing.

> I was working on an adult psychiatric unit one weekend when the nursing administrator telephoned me to say that a patient I had previously worked with had been admitted on one of the other units. The administrator was concerned that the patient, a well-developed young male, was not speaking to anyone, and they really didn't know what was going on with him. She asked if I would come and speak with him and build on our previous relationship. I recognized the patient's name and said that I would come.
>
> When I arrived, the patient was in his room with the door opened. I greeted him. He seemed to recognize me, and I stepped into the room, leaving the door open. To my surprise, he immediately moved to the door, shut it, and silently stood in front of it, staring at me. My heart started to pound, and I could feel my stomach tightening. I became aware that the patient was in tenuous touch with reality, and

I became very concerned for my safety. Something in my own physical responsiveness in my gut brought me back to our previous encounter. During that time I had identified gastrointestinal symptoms in the patient that resulted in his emergency treatment for a perforated ulcer, which probably helped save his life. Because I knew that one of his symptoms was paranoia, I used this recollection to reconnect with the patient and reassure him that I wanted to help, not hurt, him. As he continued to stare, he walked away from the door and placed himself on the opposite wall, leaving a clear path to the door. I looked at him, said thank you, and slowly left the room. He closed the door. My heart sank as the staff on the unit began to discuss how to treat this patient who was having an acute exacerbation of symptoms related to paranoid schizophrenia.

This experience serves as a reminder that when a nurse offers an authentic presence to a patient, the patient somehow apprehends the gesture and responds to the human connection offered.

Practical Wisdom

Aristotle defines practical wisdom as a "true and reasoned state or capacity to act with regard to the things that are good or bad for humankind" (350 BC, Book VI, 5). Practical wisdom is the golden thread that is interwoven throughout all nursing activities and may be distinguished by its deliberative and purposive qualities. That is, it is marked by a "thinking about" that leads to an elaboration of the essential nature of the nursing occasion in which a nurse is occupied. Practical wisdom enhances the application of scientific and other forms of knowledge by bringing into the equation of patient care concern for, and attendance to, aspects of human affairs that fall outside the boundaries of medical and technical competence. Practical wisdom relates to such aspects of human affairs as morality, ethics, dignity, respect, humility, and spirituality. These and other aspects of human affairs relate not only to patients but also to families, caregivers, other health-care professionals, and nurses.

The experience with the psychiatric patient, given above, and the following experience of a nurse practitioner interacting with an adolescent offer examples of practical wisdom, along with concern and pathic touch. Each of these examples shows how these concepts are intricately related and tightly woven into a tapestry of human centered care.

The following excerpt comes from an interview with a nurse practitioner who specializes in pediatrics:

In my practice I have to think constantly about what I am doing in order to improvise ways to try to accomplish what needs to be done with my patients. That even comes up with something as simple as taking clothes off or not. I had a patient the other day, a preadolescent, almost 11 years old. She knows me a little bit. My assistant came back and said to me, "She's crying, absolutely crying in the waiting room saying, 'I'm not doing this.'" And I sat down with the mother, and she said, "I've got to tell you. There's enough going on with her, I'm sure, in her life, but for some reason she is freaked about this today. Part of it is I didn't tell her we were coming. I forgot." I said, "Okay, I appreciate it. But don't worry, I'll work with her." And, lo and behold, when the patient got in the room, she did not want her mother in the room. They're always given that option at a certain age. So that was probably the best thing, in this case, that could have happened. Because she got over whatever she had going on. And we really had a very, very good exam and exchange.

The tears dried up; she was smiling, and she had all her clothes on. I walked in, and I said, "Hi, Danielle. How are you doing?" And she was kind of smiling. I said to her, "So I understand this wasn't exactly what you had in mind this afternoon. Sorry about that." I just sort of accepted that she felt uneasy. Immediately I could see her relax. You know, her face skin loosened. I think she appreciated that I accepted that. She knew her mother was talking to me about how she felt about the exam, and I didn't hide it. Beyond that, she was very open with me.

I just decided to go forward now. She didn't look too freaked out. So, again, I think it's something I read in her facial expression and how she was talking to me and she was animated and pretty happy. I think I really was tuned in. I just said, "I guess I understand that you weren't particularly thrilled having me do a vaginal exam today. But, you know what—I'm going to let that go for today. I'm going to allow you that privacy today, but, you know, I do need to do it sometime. That is a part of your exams, and these are the reasons why." And I said, "Next year I'm going to remind you that you're another year older, and it's going to be important to get through that part of the exam." It was helpful to know in advance that she was flipped out, but I think on the other hand, it could have gone the other way.

Some parents come in with a tremendous number of issues. And I am very careful to make sure, first of all, that they have the chance to talk to me about it. So I am very flexible. Sometimes they're a lot more concerned about an issue than I am. So I just have to be careful to allow them to let me know what it is about their child that they are concerned about. And with some parents they're very happy to hear that I think the child is perfectly fine. Sometimes, while I might not be so concerned, the parent really wants more services and more interaction to just sort out the problem. It's just something about the mother's level of anxiety that she expresses about the problem that tells me how to proceed.

So I do learn about different parents, and I do learn from the way they ask questions; the content of their questions; the way they interact with their children. I see a lot of newborns. When the parents walk in the room with the baby, I immediately can tell how anxious they are and how comfortable they are with a newborn. And so I actually do behave differently, depending on how anxious they are. And you know what, the baby acts differently. I have those great young parents that are bouncing the baby around, and they don't have a million questions. I just can tell they're a little bit more relaxed. And others, I can tell, are going to need a little bit more direction and instruction and reassurance that the baby's doing well.

The conceptual framework of human centered nursing interweaves the concepts of pathic touch, concern, and practical wisdom. These concepts and their interrelationships provide a structure of human centered nursing that serves to explain and clarify the phenomenon of human centered caring. The structure of human centered nursing identifies the pathic touch as the dynamic that facilitates the connection to the patient. This connection offers possibilities for becoming aware of the concerns of the patient in concert with the concerns of the nurse. Through practical wisdom, the nurse complements her scientific knowledge and life experiences with a pathic understanding of her patient, incorporating moral, ethical, and spiritual aspects in a dignified and respectful manner.

REFERENCES

Alford, R. (1998). *The craft of inquiry: Theories, methods, evidence.* New York: Oxford University Press.

Aristotle. (350 BC). *Nicomachean ethics,* trans. Ross WD. Accessed March 23, 2003. Available at http://classics.mit.edu//Aristotle/nicomachaen.html

Heidegger, M. (1927/1962). *Being and time,* trans. J. Macquarrie & E. Robinson. San Francisco: Harper & Row.

Schutz, A. (1970). *On phenomenology and social relations: Selected writings.* Chicago: University of Chicago Press.

van Manen, M. (1999). The pathic nature of inquiry and nursing. In I. Madjar & J. Walton, eds., *Nursing and the experience of illness: Phenomenology in practice* (pp 17–35). London: Routledge.

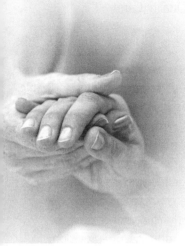

Chapter 5

Methodological Topics in Human Centered Nursing

Through human centered nursing, nurses may discover and participate in the essential nature of nursing. In seeking the essential nature of nursing, nurses require a methodology that offers possibilities for discovering and illuminating the fundamental truths that underlie the nature of nursing. Such a methodology provides direct insight into the values and meanings that define the nursing act and a way to articulate these values and meanings as they occur in nursing occasions. The choice for accomplishing this task is the phenomenological method of inquiry, referred to as a search for meaning or a search for the essential nature of some phenomenon (Merleau-Ponty, 1962).

This chapter briefly explores the phenomenological method. Then it provides a plan for integrating the phenomenological method of inquiry into students' activities in the classroom and/or clinic. The exercise provided is part of the humanistic teaching method, which educators may include as part of their pedagogical strategy. Student observations and reflections are included to help illustrate the method and provide outcomes of the process in the classroom setting. The exercise is presented in the standard lesson plan format of: purpose, activities, expected outcomes, and observed outcomes.

Phenomenological Inquiry Generally

The phenomenological method is the method of choice rather than the logical/deductive/statistical methods of science, like those based on hypothesis testing, decision analysis, and causal modeling. These latter methods require computation and/or logical deduction of quantitative (numerical and symbolic) variables and seek rational explanations and predictions based on mathematically and logically derived relationships in the data. These data-based methods of analysis do not yield the richest result when inquiring into phenomena that occur during nursing occasions. They do not yield the meanings and values underpinning the nursing experience (Alford, 1998; Paterson and Zderad, 1976). Furthermore, and most importantly, these methods do not offer a process of inquiry that is enjoyable, enlightening, and inspiring and that affords the possibility for the development of self.

As Edgar Schein (2006) eloquently stated:

> As I think about graduate training and the models of the professoriate that I see reflected in many of my colleagues, I get a sense of discouragement and unreality. There is something very limiting and depressing in the traditional model of science with its emphasis on precision, operational definitions, the hypothetical-deductive method, quantification, statistical manipulation, and deadly dry reporting [of generally only positive results].

By contrast, the phenomenological method is expansive and discovery-oriented. It is satisfying for students and practicing nurses alike to be able to reflect on an experience and be uplifted by the realization that they have discovered the true meaning of that experience and how that meaning fits in with the totality of their systems of beliefs and daily practice of nursing. This method often inspires nurses to discover truths about why they became or remain nurses and helps them to recapture the excitement of making a difference in the lives of others.

The road that leads to the truths of nursing is traveled via phenomenological reflection on experiences. The journey holds a promise to come to know and understand oneself, to know and understand others, and to gain insight into the nature of nursing. In this way, what becomes known to each nurse can be integrated into the nursing practice of that nurse and others with whom she interacts in her community.

Nurses and students are urged to analyze phenomenological reflections within the context of aspects of human centered nursing practice. A procedure and examples for this task are given below. In that way, nurses may illuminate the essential nature of the various fields of concern that define and differentiate the life worlds they occupy at a given moment in time. Such worlds include, for example, the world of the nurse, the world of the mother or father, the world of the teacher, and the world of the student.

The technique of phenomenological reflection is distinct from reflection as looking back, or reviewing, what was done in a particular situation in order to improve nursing quality or productivity. Phenomenological reflection is concerned with revealing "meanings" of experiences rather than details of particular nursing acts. It is done within some form of theoretical or conceptual framework as well as within definite disciplinary and phenomenal contexts that serve to draw attention to a particular horizon of wonderment.

The previous chapter articulated the theoretical and conceptual frameworks of human centered nursing. This somewhat amorphous field of investigation keeps attention focused on immediate areas of concern and the search for truths within that framework. Because the subject here is human nature, other theoretical/conceptual frameworks may be similar to and have similar constitutive attributes as others. Some possible conceptual frameworks include political theory, social theory, and religious theory. For instance, human centered nursing is concerned with truths of human interactions and relationships that offer possibilities for each person to become more because of the encounter. "Becoming more" means enhancement of self-actualizing potential. On the other hand, in an investigation based on political theory, the theoretical and conceptual attributes are ideology, oratory, campaign methodologies, appointments, and cronyism. Political theory may focus on social interaction of individuals and groups to the extent that they satisfy the requirements of an orderly state within the confines of laws and other guidelines for social interactions.

The phenomenal context includes particular events from which empirical evidence or observations are observed. For example, in human centered nursing, nurses interact with patients, teachers interact with students, nurses interact with families, and nurses interact with other nurses and other health-care professionals, during which particular moments of experience occur. Focusing the dialogue and observations on a particular phenomenon, rather than roaming about, reduces the potential for being distracted by introducing too many different ideas and perspectives into the dialogue.

Once learned, the method of phenomenological inquiry can be used to enhance other aspects of nurses' lives beyond the nurse/patient dialogue. Paterson and Zderad have used the method of phenomenological reflection on experiences in situations outside of nursing. Paterson and Zderad spoke about how phenomenological inquiry helped them think about and get through many of the changes and difficulties of their careers and the crisis of having to do something else (personal conversation, 2001). A student also reported:

> Many positive changes have started in my life in conjunction with phenomenological inquiry. I am learning. I am growing. I have started applying the reflection techniques in my daily practices. I have gained awareness of

the effect of my reactions on my son primarily and on other people. I started my own personal journal aside from the one required for class.

Integrating the Phenomenological Method

This exercise demonstrates a pedagogical strategy used by educators applying the humanistic teaching method.

Purpose of the Exercise

The purpose of the exercise is to introduce students to the method of phenomenological inquiry in order to (1) bring out meanings embedded in their experiences, so that (2) they will gain insight into human responses to health-care situations. Each engagement in phenomenological inquiry offers possibilities to enrich their acquired experiential wisdom and use that wisdom in the service of their patients. Furthermore, the method of phenomenological inquiry can take nurses beyond the fields of nursing concerns by engendering possibilities for becoming more as persons within the frameworks of all of their life's activities and relationships. Simply stated, the phenomenological method of inquiry provides a method of inquiring into the fundamental values and meanings that contribute to each person's level of self-actualization (Box 5–1).

Exercise Activities

Each lesson introduces and focuses on particular areas of study—clinical or theoretical, or both—that have significance for nursing occasions. Examples include humanism, existentialism, phenomenology, pathic touch, concern, practical wisdom, culture, ethics, communications, group dynamics, critical thinking, and conflict resolution. These points of emphasis are either the primary topic in a fundamentals or introductory course or embedded in topical courses such as pediatrics, psychiatric-mental health, and emergency care. These points of emphasis are interrelated by reason of overlapping theoretical or conceptual constituents directed at the well-being of a whole person rather than taken in the isolated abstract. Directing attention to the well-being of the whole person is a distinguishing characteristic of nursing. Nurses focus on health-related concerns of patients as part of the condition of a whole person instead of examining only the symptoms related to particular ailments separate and distinct from the person occupied with them. Therefore, while highlighting a particular point or points in the context of a nursing occasion, other relevant aspects of nursing are always present to some extent.

Box 5–1 | Self-Actualization as Conceptualized in Human Centered Nursing

1. Self-actualization is a process of emotional and moral development that contributes to the more-being and well-being of each individual. The self-actualizing nurse is one who is engaged in the process of becoming true to herself and to those with whom she goes through life's experiences.

2. Self-actualizing nurses: (a) place value on what they do as nurses and nursing as a profession; (b) examine their own nursing experiences in order to reveal and illuminate the essential aspects of those experiences, bringing those essential aspects into current consciousness; (c) through reflection and examination of their experiences of being in the world and their world of nursing, reveal and illuminate the essential values and meanings that these experiences hold for them; (d) express values and meanings that are internally generated, not externally imposed; (e) manifest these important values and meanings through complementary behaviors; in both demeanor and actions; (f) learn to know themselves and, through that, know others.

3. The qualities observed in the self-actualizing nurse are as follows: (a) the self-actualizing nurse presents with competence and confidence; (b) the attitude of the self-actualizing nurse radiates positively to her patients, families, coworkers, and community; (c) the self-actualizing nurse is a locus for high-quality care and patient satisfaction; (d) the self-actualizing nurse, by her mere "presence," makes a difference in the lives of everyone she encounters.

4. Self-actualization, once experienced, becomes a continuous process of always striving to develop and achieve higher levels of excellence and gratification.

(Boeree, G., 2004; Paterson and Zderad, 1976)

Overview

Specifically, instructors should present articles and case studies selected from the scholarly nursing literature that illustrate the issue or issues being discussed. Then students participate in open discussions in which they draw on their own experiences.

These situations may concern professional, intimate, or casual relationships with patients, health-care professionals, fellow students and teachers, or family members, friends, and acquaintances.

Students bring into these discussions their own values, meanings, perceptions of the situation, and theoretical interpretations, which may agree or conflict with those of patients, families, or institutions. Each student tends to color the situation somewhat differently by virtue of his personal background and acquired experiential wisdom. Each student is also required to place the entire situation in the context of professional practice, paying particular attention to the nurse's social policy statement and code of ethics, patient's bill of rights, and professional and legal standards. As a follow-up to the material presented and discussed in class, students are required to write self-reflections on their interactions with patients or in response to classroom activities, which they may share in open class presentations. These sharing activities make students aware of the similarities and differences of perceptions among their peers and stimulate the desire to discuss these in open dialogue.

Literature and Reflections

Students are presented with a variety of selections from the literature that engage them in the process of phenomenological inquiry and excite their awareness of the diverse possibilities for reflection. Sources of selections include scholarly papers, books, videos, movie clips, and documentaries. Works of art, particularly poetry, illustrate the value of the aesthetic in conveying the essential nature of nursing as well as the essential nature of life in general. Observe the power that a work of art has in conveying such meaning in the reflections of four students who responded to the film, *What Do You See, Nurse?* (McCormick, 1980), which is a dramatization of "A Crabbit Old Woman," a poem written by a patient at Ashludie Hospital near Dunde, England. After the woman died in the geriatric ward of the hospital, this poem was found among her possessions. Copies were made for all the nurses in the hospital. Addressed to the nurses who surrounded the woman in her last days, this poem cries for recognition of a common humanity:

What do you see, nurse...what do you see?

Are you thinking—when you look at me:

"A crabbit old woman, not very wise;

Uncertain of habit with far-away eyes,

Who dribbles her food and makes no reply

When you say in a loud voice 'I do wish you'd try.'"

Who seems not to notice the things that you do

And forever is losing a stocking or shoe;

Who, resisting or not, lets you do as you will

With bathing and feeding, the long day to fill.

Is that what you're thinking, is that what you see?

Then open your eyes, nurse. You're not looking at me!

I'll tell you who I am as I sit here so still.

As I move at your bidding, eat at your will:

—I'm a small child often with a father and mother,

Brothers and sisters who love one another;

—A young girl of sixteen with wings on her feet,

Dreaming that soon a love she'll meet;

—A bride at twenty, my heart gives a leap,

Remembering the vows that I promised to keep;

—At twenty-five now I have young of my own

Who need me to build a secure, happy home.

As we were discussing family in class last week, I felt that she was my family. She felt so close and valued to the staff that she said she will miss us. The definition of family doesn't only mean someone who we live with by birth because we as nurses touch our patient's lives so much each day that they feel that we are their family.

Expected Outcomes

Following are expected outcomes of the exercise:

- Students will demonstrate their ability and willingness to implement phenomenological inquiry into their thinking and dialogues about the values and meanings of their nursing experiences.
- All the nurses will recognize opportunities to become more as people and be inspired to help others to become more, regardless of the situation in which they find themselves.
- Lessons will come alive for students as they explore both theoretical and practical aspects of issues that arise during nursing occasions.
- Students will become astute at defining and describing each issue from both a theoretical and practical standpoint as well as being able to determine the congruency of the particular nursing occasion with their own sets of values and meanings.
- By sharing their experiences in open discussions with the class, students will become aware of the unpredictability of and many possibilities for differing human responses to nursing situations.
- Students will integrate and expand the ideas discovered in the lessons while engaging in interactions and relationships with patients and health-care professionals.

Observed Outcomes

The observed outcomes provide the teacher and student with a way of evaluating the learning of each student and the effectiveness of the pedagogical strategies being employed. Outcomes also assess the extent to which each student's learning offers possibilities to enhance the quality of nurse-patient relationships and, by extension, the quality of patient care.

The following excerpts from students' writings give testimony to what they learned about themselves by engaging in phenomenological inquiry and how what they learned affected their nursing activities. These examples of students' writings demonstrate the potential for enhancing learning, high-quality patient care, and personal and professional growth and satisfaction through the humanistic teaching method. Each of these anecdotes is given with a topical header that signals the conceptual basis of each student's commentary. They have been left intact and unedited intentionally in order to retain authenticity.

On Phenomenological Reflection as a Way of Valuing Nursing Experiences

I have gained a theoretical and practical grounding for my intuition about what it means to be a nurse and a means of examining the values and meanings of my own nursing activities. Reflecting on my nursing experiences took me on a journey full of insights. I looked back at my nursing career with new eyes. Reflecting on my nursing experiences opened my mind to the many dimensions of treating a patient as a human being. Too often I was taken into the mechanical and technical aspect of nursing. My interrelationships with the patient would be sometimes limited to the "I" and "it." With new knowledge I strive to ensure that I live my nursing career to its fullest, focusing on each patient as a whole and unique individual.

Reflecting on and analyzing my experiences adds more sense to my nursing practice, helps me to validate it. I feel grounded, for I can go back to my experiences and retrieve valuable information that helps me grow. I seek more to explore and to understand the meanings for my nursing practice. I hope to be able to help my patients toward more being while I am becoming more as a person.

Integrating Theory Into Practice

While reviewing and studying for today's exam, I had the strange feeling that pieces from my learning were falling into place. Humanism is such a broad concept. To take just a small grasp of it would be a crime. In reality everything in life is simple yet large enough that it embraces more than just one aspect. As a health professional, it is so important to evaluate and define my limits in order to know what I can and cannot do. More important is to stop and listen, vital to understand the "other" in a larger context. Or is it that all these aspects are of equal importance? As I mentioned many pieces started falling in place...I became aware that a certain level of internal maturation had occurred since day one. In other words the cake was baked. I was so excited, finally in the palm of my hands I was starting to hold and appreciate my efforts. I am more than grateful for the many instructors that gave me knowledge and the tools necessary for me to be where I am. I am grateful for the freedom to decide what to do with this vast material. I am grateful because simple actions lead me through the right way. What also amazed me was that I was applying concepts learned here in many other facets of my life. Once again I feel I am in the right place at the right time.

On Self-Actualization

In all my studies in nursing none have been as educative for me as the experience of this class. I have been empowered and energized. The positive impact on me cannot be overstated and I know and believe that all the patients I cared for must have gained enormously from my recent improvement in my nursing proficiency. Even my colleagues recognize the difference in me and give me positive comments. I am reminded of what it means to be a nurse and the reasons I became a nurse in the first place. I was considering quitting nursing but I have gotten fresh insight into what nursing is all about and I have become determined to stay on as a nurse. I also learned how to examine my nursing experiences to bring forward those aspects of nursing that I value.

Making Choices—Finding One's Self

I had a patient who was dying, alone in her room, while at the same time my supervisor was demanding that I attend a meeting about administrative details. My supervisor said, "You go ahead and do what you want. What do you want to do?" I said, "I am going to sit with the patient and hold her hand." I decided that the priorities in that institution were not consistent with my own and I subsequently quit that job and found another hospital more amenable to my style of patient care.

Summary

This chapter introduced and presented the phenomenological method of inquiry as the preferred research method for nurses who wish to explore and evaluate their nursing experiences, derive values and meanings for those experiences, and enable self-actualization and personal and professional growth and satisfaction. The chapter explored advantages of the phenomenological method and addressed the process of how to implement it into the classroom.

REFERENCES

Alford, R. (1998). *The craft of inquiry: Theories, methods, evidence.* New York: Oxford University Press.

Boeree, G. (2004). *Abraham Maslow.* Accessed March 18, 2008, from http://webspace.ship.edu/cgboer/maslow.html

McCormick, P. (1980). *What do you see, nurse?* A film by McCormick Educational Technology Center: Union, Mo.

Merleau-Ponty, M. (1962). *Phenomenology of perception*, trans. C. Smith. New York: Routledge & Kegan Paul.

Paterson, J., & Zderad, L. (1976). *Humanistic nursing.* New York: Wiley.

Schein, E. (2006). *The academic as artist: Personal and professional roots.* Retrieved February 23, 2006, from www.edschein.com

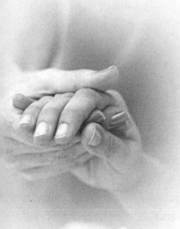

Chapter 6

Implementing the Phenomenological Method of Inquiry in Nursing Research

T
his chapter elaborates on the steps involved in implementing the phenomenological method of inquiry, including:

Stating a research question of interest (see comment at end)

Acquiring data

Deriving and analyzing concepts

Analyzing the data

Presenting results or findings.

This chapter includes three examples of how to implement phenomenological research. Students, teachers, and researchers may adapt these examples to the varied research opportunities that arise in nursing scholarship.

The first example is a template for implementing the phenomenological method of inquiry nuanced for nursing research, which is extrapolated from an article "Phenomenology: To Wonder and Search for Meaning" (Kleiman [2004b]). The second example is based on Paterson's and Zderad's implementation of phenomenology. Nurses are shown how to derive and renew their own meanings and values for nursing and share them with others.

The final example is a group project for experienced nurses in which participants become familiar with the reflective process of phenomenology. Reflection on experiences is used as a way to reaffirm one's reasons for becoming and remaining a nurse and strengthening participation in the community of nurses. One reward for this effort is a higher level of self-actualization in the attainment of personal and professional growth.

Phenomenological Method Nuanced for Nursing Research

This first example speaks to the student or researcher who is engaged in or intending to become engaged in phenomenological nursing research.

During an evening in Paris, Raymond Aron, a distinguished sociologist, philosopher, historian, and journalist, was drinking with Jean-Paul Sartre and Simone de Beauvoir, Sartre's longtime companion, lover, and collaborator. Aron mentioned Husserl's new method of phenomenology, which presented Sartre with the tool he had been searching for in order to formulate and communicate his thoughts. Aron used a beer mug to illustrate phenomenology, discussing the mug's properties and essence (Wyatt, 2003).

What piqued Sartre's interest was Husserl's formulation of a method of inquiry that would enable him to set aside the highly esoteric and abstract musings of philosophical exhortations. Sartre was excited by the prospect of being able to investigate and describe the presence of any phenomenon given to consciousness, precisely as it is experienced, and come to understand the phenomenon in terms of the meaning that it had for the experiencing subject. In simple terms, he liked the idea of examining what comes into a person's current consciousness or awareness and what the meaning of that awareness is for the beholder (Wyatt, 2003). Husserl (1913) coined the precept *zu den Sachen selbst* (toward or back to the things themselves) to designate the focal point of his phenomenological inquiry.

The Basic Task

When a researcher inquires into the nature of an experience, the primary task is to discover and elucidate the meanings that underlie that experience (Merleau-Ponty, 1962). The meanings of interest are those that are always present in the occurrence or recurrence of a particular experience and serve as identifying characteristics of that experience (Giorgi, 1997, 2003). For example, when one person reaches out to help another who is in need, that reaching out has some meaning or meanings for each person. The meanings could be based on a fundamental nature of human beings toward each other; a familial, moral, ethical, or community obligation; a spiritual mandate of some kind; or some combination thereof. Meanings may be thought of as the "why" a particular experience unfolds for a person or persons in the manner that it does and are explanatory rather than numerically specifiable. Phenomenology is interested in how the nature of certain nursing experiences can be understood through nurses' reflective descriptions of what is going on during nursing occasions.

Design Considerations for a Phenomenological Inquiry

The language of phenomenology, while precise within the method, does not use terms commonly heard in everyday conversation. Two terms ubiquitous within phenomenology need clarification. The first is "essence" and its cognates; for example, essential and essentiality. In everyday life pursuits, human beings strive toward some ideal or perfection that could be legitimately called essential to their mode of being-in-the-world, and yet the term essence can be troublesome. Merleau-Ponty (1962) pointed out that phenomenology is the study of essences; all problems amount to finding definitions of essences; the essence serves to identify an experience as what it is.

The second term is "lived experience." Lived experiences are those experiences that reveal the immediate, pre-reflective consciousness an individual has regarding events in which that individual has participated. Individuals use such lived experiences as the basis for recalling how they lived through the event, thereby bringing them into current consciousness.

Formulating the Research Question

Going to the "thing itself" as a starting point for discovery and articulation of meanings of lived experiences helps in the formulation of a research question. The research question succinctly defines what the research, study, or inquiry is asking about. The research question and its implicit method of analysis are always preceded by an explicit identification of the subject or phenomenon of interest. According to Alford (1998), the research question for any project entails both an empirical and a theoretical component.

In the paradigm of phenomenological inquiry, the generic empirical question is, "What are the essential meanings of any phenomena—human behavior, lived experience, or activity—that come into the consciousness of, and are described by, the participants in the study?" The generic theoretical question is, "What is the structure, gleaned from the raw data (i.e., the participants' descriptions), that articulates the nature or meaning of the phenomenon under study?"

Excerpts supporting the following discussion are from a research report on the essential nature of nurses' experiences interacting with their patients (Kleiman, 2004a). For example, the following research question was defined to reflect the author's interest in the meanings that nurses assign to their interactions with patients: What is the nature of nurses' lived experiences interacting with patients? The empirical question was: What are the essential meanings of nurse/patient interactions brought into current consciousness and given in nurses' descriptions of their experiences? The theoretical question was: "What is the structure, gleaned from the essential meanings, of nurses' experiences interacting with patients?

Sample and Method of Selection

Once the research question is stipulated, it is important to determine the type of sample and number of participants that will lend insight into the phenomena under study. How many participants are necessary to obtain rich data descriptions in a particular study? A sampling technique that is particularly suited to phenomenological inquiry is the snowball, purposive sampling method. Using this method, the researcher adds participants until the needed data requirements are met, ordinarily signaled by obvious redundancy. This usually ranges from one to a maximum of approximately ten participants for phenomenological research (Giorgi, 2003).

In the research report, there were six participants. Some redundancies were experienced after the third participant was interviewed. Examples of redundancies included direct patient contact, time with patients and families, and attentive and empathic attitude. These responses appeared in all three cases, giving a feeling for redundancy. Even with three more participants, new aspects of patient interaction did not seem to be forthcoming, thereby conveying the feeling of redundancy or "enough." The researcher is cautioned, however, not to stop arbitrarily at some point but to go on a little further in search of new revelations.

Theoretical Design Constructs

What are the necessary theoretical design constructs for a method to qualify as phenomenological in a descriptive, Husserlian sense? How were these design constructs implemented in the research report? The design constructs are:

1. Concrete description(s) of the phenomenon under study as present to the participant(s)
2. Analysis within the attitude of the phenomenological reduction
3. Discovery and elucidation of the essential meanings for a context (Giorgi, 1997, 2003).

Note that the design constructs are the minimum required for a study to be considered phenomenology. These are the higher-level constructs. The next section goes through the process step by step with more detail. These steps are not "mandated" but are necessary according to the author, and may be altered by another researcher.

Concrete Descriptions of the Phenomenon of Interest

The first step in collecting data is to get descriptions of lived experiences from the participants. These descriptions should be as free from generalizations and abstractions as possible. To observe the phenomenon as presented by participants, the researcher puts aside all preconceived ideas, enters into a relationship of dialogic openness, and is ready to allow the participant to speak and ready to listen (Palmer, 1999; Parse, 2003; Paterson & Zderad, 1976). This proffered readiness to listen inspires participants to relate what presents itself to their consciousness in the immediate situation. Openness of this type is facilitated by conducting the interviews in an environment that is comfortable for the participant, even if the researcher may not consider the location ideal. For example, one nurse who participated in the cited research study chose to meet in a café where jazz was playing in the background. Although initially concerned about background noise and privacy, the researcher soon became aware through the nurse's demeanor that she was relaxed, open, and truly engaged in the direct interview process.

Through direct face-to-face meetings, the researcher sees the nuances of the participant's experiences, conveyed through facial expressions, blushing, gestures, tears, sounds, silences, and other vocal dynamics. The researcher's reflective experiences of the nuances of the participant's descriptions, derived from the face-to-face encounter, come to life during the analysis. The further away from the concrete, face-to-face descriptions a researcher gets, the more abstract the analysis will be and the less likely that it will convey the meaning intended by the participant at that time (Schutz, 1970). Therefore, the person who conducts the interview gets the richest appreciation of the descriptions rendered in the interviews and should, whenever possible, also do the analysis.

The descriptions of the phenomenon are elicited through open-ended, unstructured interviews, which are recorded for analysis. The questions are intended to prompt the participant but avoid any tendency to guide the response. For example, in the research study the opening question was, "Tell me about an experience you had interacting with a patient" or some variation.

Next, the researcher reads through the interviews to get a global sense of the whole. The global sense is important for determining how the parts might be constituted, which is detailed in the next step. The global sense relates to an overall grasp that, as a whole, the description seems to be a cogent representation of the participant's experience interacting with patients and the meanings those interactions bring to mind. Even the alert researcher can sometimes be misled by the interesting but extraneous intellectualizations of a participant that do not describe the participant's reflection on what she was experiencing. The global reading will bring this to light, affirming or discrediting the relevance of the data for a particular study. To achieve maximum openness, the reading takes place within the attitude of the phenomenological reduction, defined as follows.

Phenomenological Reduction

Phenomenological reduction requires stepwise implementation of two devices: bracketing and withholding the existential index.

Bracketing

Bracketing, or withholding prior knowledge of the phenomenon under study, is done in order that the researcher may take the experience precisely as it is described. The purpose is to try to assume an attentive and naïve openness to descriptions of phenomena, an uncertainty about what is to come, and a willingness to wonder about the experiences being brought to presence in the descriptions of the participants. Theorizing, conceptualizing, labeling, and categorizing according to what is already known engender a sense of complacency and comfort, depriving the researcher of the excitement of discovering the unknown about the lived experiences being studied.

The process of preparing oneself to enter the experience in wonder deserves full attention. The researcher must identify his biases and presuppositions and must be open to the existence of many possibilities for experiencing a phenomenon. In the cited study, the researcher, a nurse with 20 years of nursing and psychotherapy experience, had to withhold any presuppositions about the nature and progression of the interaction process being described. In preparation for doing the interviews and subsequent analysis of the data, the researcher dialogued with colleagues who questioned and brought forward the researcher's awareness of her previous knowledge, experience, and beliefs. In addition, the researcher was challenged by these colleagues to be open to the possibility of something that is yet unknown. An example of this process can be gleaned from the Kitchen Dialogues with Paterson and Zderad in Chapter 3.

Withholding the Existential Index

Withholding the existential index involves considering what is given, precisely as it is given, as presence or phenomenon (Giorgi, 1997, 2003). One says that an object presents itself as such and such, rather than saying that an object is such and such, regardless of how obvious it is. Therefore, after observing a table—a real table—a researcher, within the attitude of phenomenological reduction, says, "The table presents itself to me as a really existing table." This is more rigorous than saying, "It is a real table." Withholding the existential index facilitates the analysis of phenomena that are not easily recognized as particular "objects," such as emotions or values or experiences.

Bracketing and withholding the existential index complement each other. Their use strengthens the analysis. The researcher does not forget all possible past knowledge, but holds in abeyance, or brackets, all past knowledge of the phenomena that may influence her perception or originality in the present situation.

Discriminate Meaning Units

Review the interviews again more slowly in order to divide them into "meaning units." A meaning unit may be words spoken by the participant that have a definite theme or relationship or meaning among them. Now in the course of everyday conversation—that in which the interviews are conducted—people naturally shift from one detail or theme to another, even though the whole story has some cohesive structure. When the researcher experiences a shift in meaning in the words of the participant, the shift is acknowledged and highlighted.

Consider this example that appeared in the cited research report. A nurse concerned with a patient's obesity said, "Because she was an accountant, I said to her, if somebody was spending all his money in his business and not balancing his checkbook, that would be considered sort of a dangerous behavior, and she agreed that it would be." In the next sentence, the same nurse, demonstrating an obvious shift of the conversation said, "Physicians for the most part don't spend the time it takes to work with patients that they think are uncooperative."

A discrimination of all similar shifts in meaning is applied to all the statements in the interview. In this brief example, the shift in direction occurred rapidly, from one sentence to another. Each meaning unit may include multiple sentences, paragraphs, or even pages, however, and the shifts may be more subtle. Meaning units having similar focus or content are integrated in order to clarify the sense of the participant's descriptions. For example:

- "I'm here."/"I'll be here."/"I'm still here."
- "I tell them I'm available and that they can call me."/"I tell [my patients] that I'm here for them if they need to talk about it."

Relevance for the Phenomenon of Interest

The meaning units are reviewed for relevance to the phenomenon of interest. Here again the analysis must maintain its focus. To avoid a radical redirection of the analysis toward a particular goal or result, take caution to avoid deciding arbitrarily that a particular statement is not relevant. Rigorous phenomenological technique requires accounting for all the data and does not allow for arbitrarily ignoring or erasing a particular statement. If you encounter a statement that seems to be irrelevant, mark it as such, and continue on. An example of such a statement is: "I am very angry at them. I feel really betrayed by my professional organization, you know all this carrying on about the doctor doing this and doing that, but meanwhile it is my professional organization that causes me problems." Recall that in the research study, the research question was focused on the essential nature of nurses interacting with patients. The shift to relationships with professional organizations is not relevant to the phenomenon of interest in this context.

Disciplinary Perspective

The researcher remains faithful to the disciplinary perspective of nursing, consistent with the study requirements. It is legitimate to impose a disciplinary perspective of, for example, sociology, psychology, anthropology, or pedagogy to nursing studies. Once established, however, the disciplinary perspective does not change. In the example above, in which a nurse working with a patient who had been an accountant uses a metaphor of financial capriciousness to express concern about the patient's disregard for the effects of obesity on physical health, the meaning unit is analyzed properly from the disciplinary perspective of nursing because the study is not interested in financial capriciousness or stability. The nurse uses the metaphor to get the obesity point across to the patient and is interested in her personal rather than financial health.

Finding Essential Meanings and Gleaning the General Structure

In compliance with the third element of phenomenological design constructs, the next step is to discover and elucidate the essential meanings for the experiences of each nurse interacting with her patients. The discriminated meaning units derived from each nurse's experiences are integrated and compared and contrasted. Themes are identified and grouped together, keeping within the boundaries of the disciplinary perspective. This step allows some procedural flexibility on the part of the researcher. In the research study, all of the meaning units from all of the participants were integrated into one construct for analysis. Alternatively, a construct could have been developed for each participant, and then all constructs would be integrated.

Next, the process of free imaginative variation is employed by removing and replacing each meaning unit in turn in order to determine which of the meaning units is essential for, and constitutive of, a fixed identity for the phenomenon under study. For example, being present to patients in an open and attentive manner was determined to be an essential property or meaning of nurses' interactions with patients. If this property or meaning was removed, the phenomenon under study would lose its identity as defined in the experiences of the nurse participants. What is an essential property? A really simple analogy that hints at the meaning of essential property or meaning is the chocolate in a chocolate cake. If we take away the chocolate from a chocolate cake, we would not be able to identify the "thing" as a chocolate cake.

By using the device of free imaginative variation, a particular phenomenon (experiences of nurses) may be subjected to every imaginable variation among its meaning units to see how far it can be stretched before it loses its identity. Meanings that have no effect on the identity of a particular phenomenon are not considered essential to that phenomenon. An example of a meaning unit not essential to the phenomenon of interest was offered by a participant in the cited research report who advocated social and political activism in her interactions with patients: "I tell them that it's a political issue. It's the tenor of the political climate in the United States today. So if you think it is important, you have to vote, and you have to act. Your health is not something idle. Your health is social, political, familial; it has everything to do with the environment, with society." Although advocating social and political activism is a part of this nurse's demeanor and way of life, that particular meaning was not necessary to the identity of the phenomenon under study. Keep in mind that although meaning units are introduced into the domain of interest by nurses, it is not the nurses who are under inquiry; it is the phenomenon that is evidenced in the descriptions of their experiences. In other words, a researcher is not using phenomenological method until he starts analyzing and talking about the phenomenon and not the people participating in it.

Elaboration of the Findings

After going through the above processes, the researcher elaborates the findings. This includes describing the essential meanings discovered through the process of free imaginative variation and articulating a structure of the phenomenon gleaned from those discovered essential meanings and their relationships.

In the cited research report, the essential meanings of the lived experiences of nurses interacting with patients were: openness, connection, concern, respect, reciprocity, competence, time, and professional identity. These essential meanings have closely interrelated qualities and are not to be considered as discrete elements. Rather, they are complementary; in a particular situation, where one meaning has foreground presence, it is likely that more meanings will also be present. This inter-relationship of the essential meanings is illustrated in the situation in which the nurse in her interaction with the patient fosters a connection by being open to and respectful of the patient because of an overriding concern regarding a life-threatening health situation. Connection, openness, and respect are all evident, and in the foreground of this situation is concern.

On the other hand, while each essential meaning supports the fundamental meaning of the interaction, no definite measurable or specifiable relationship exists because these relationships may change with each unique nursing occasion. In another instance the essential meaning of respect may take the foreground when the nurse, through her openness, becomes aware of a cultural or religious requirement and, despite the constraints of limited time, respects the patient's need to fulfill this requirement and adjusts the treatment schedule.

The essential meanings and their qualities derived from the data in the cited research report are listed in Table 6–1. Following the table in Box 6–1 is a definition of reciprocity, one of the derived essential meanings. Examples from the reflections from several nurses in the study are also included.

Structure of the Phenomenon of Interest

The structure is the major finding pulled from a descriptive phenomenological inquiry. The researcher articulates a structure based upon the essential meanings present in the descriptions offered by participants. The structure is determined by the prior analysis and the insights obtained from the process of free imaginative variation. For the research study (Kleiman, 2004a) the structure is as follows:

> Interacting with patients is an authentic attending to health-related concerns, situated in an inter-subjective relationship (connection). The connection is engendered by a call for help from a patient to which a nurse responds. The connection flourishes in an ongoing reciprocal process of collaborative engagement of patients' health-related concerns. The connection is characterized by a constancy that prevails over time and extends beyond the direct face-to-face presences to a "presence in absence," a "being-there" for patients, even when nurses

Table 6–1 | Essential Meanings and Their Qualities (Kleiman 2004a)

Essential Meaning	Qualities
Openness	Attentive apperception, availability, readiness to listen, naïve attitude, welcoming demeanor
Connection	Authentic presence, inter-subjective dialogue, physical and/or emotional touching
Concern	Wariness and readiness to respond to phenomena confronting patient and self
Respect	Acknowledge dignity, values, self-determination
Reciprocity	The evocative interaction between nurses and patients as a manifestation of being-in-the-world with others
Competence	Effective implementation of theoretical, practical, intuitive knowledge
Time	Indistinct horizon of the possibility for nursing care, limiting all practical nursing activities
Professional identity	Advanced practice nurses, autonomous primary care providers engaged in diagnosis, medication management, directing interdisciplinary care activities, advocacy with third-party reimbursement agencies, characteristically value and spend time with patients

are corporeally absent. Notwithstanding the mood of constancy, there is an ever-present awareness of a limited amount of time to "get things done," that is, primary care, diagnosis, medication management, and advocacy and collaboration with other health-care-related services including third-party payers. Despite these constraints, the mood of inter-actions is one of non-hurried, open and attentive apperception that is couched in "listening occasions" and "presence." Due to the "intimacy" and "on-going" nature of the relationship engendered by the connection, the interactions are colored by paradoxical moods of pain and pleasure in caring for patients who are suffering.

Box 6–1 | Reciprocity

Reciprocity is a give-and-take process occurring in a complementary relationship. In nurse-patient interactions, patients respond in various ways to nurses. Unsolicited and impromptu responses from patients include fear, anger, anxiety, admiration, respect, and courage. These responses illuminate the nurse's and the patients' awareness of being-in-the-world with others and uncover the possibilities for becoming more as persons. Nurses reflected:

1. "This patient is really sick, in bad shape, but every time she comes to the floor there's a smile on her face every time she sees me. She even sends her attendant to say, 'Hello,' when she's having chemotherapy....One good thing, under the worst of conditions, if I make a difference in only one person's life for the day or the month, it really makes me feel good."

2. "You cannot help somebody else and not help yourself. I can think of several patients who, working with them, have helped me to maybe see things about myself. I've had patients who have said to me literally, 'Thank you so much, you saved my life.' Or, 'Thank you for the time you took with me.' It's nice to be acknowledged. It's nice to have people say to you, 'You did well for me, thank you.'"

3. "She gives me courage because what she's facing is very real, and she knows she might die. She knows she's 2 years ahead of the game now, and she just wants to be there for her 10-year-old."

Although nurses provide primary medical care, they define themselves as, in the first instance, "care" or "relationship" oriented, rather than "disease" or "cure" oriented. This is an important distinction that nurses make when characterizing their mode of practice.

Going Back to the Raw Data

Because the richness of phenomenology lies in the raw data, the researcher must return to the raw data descriptions to justify the articulations of both the essential meanings and the structure. The researcher reviews the raw data and must be able to point to sections in the raw data that exemplify the essential meanings defined and described. In fact, the descriptions or naming of the essential meanings should directly reflect what was said in the raw data rather than some lexicographical "fit" that may not give the appropriate nuance observed for the context in which it resides. Depending on the depth of the analysis, the astute researcher may decide to assign a name to a particular aspect of the data that expresses a particular and unique identity to the data and its context and will signal that particular meaning to the reader whenever it is encountered. For example, in the cited study, reciprocity was defined as the evocative interaction between nurses and patients as a manifestation of being-in-the-world with others. "Time" was defined as the indistinct horizon of the possibility for nursing care, limiting all practical nursing activities.

The researcher must be able to establish the accuracy of all the findings by going back to the raw data, or the findings are not valid. In fact, when the findings are submitted to the scholarly community for scrutiny or challenge, the researcher may be called upon to provide such justification for her work.

Critical Analysis of the Researcher's Work

After completing the phenomenological analysis of the data, the researcher turns to a critical analysis of the work, which includes verifying that:

- Concrete, detailed descriptions were obtained from participants
- The phenomenological reduction was assumed throughout the analysis
- Essential meanings were discovered
- A structure was articulated
- Results were confirmed by the raw data

Paterson and Zderad's Implementation of Phenomenological Method of Inquiry

Paterson and Zderad observed that, as a rule, nurses do not value their experiences. Significant awarenesses that happen during interactions with patients and colleagues remain in the background of their thinking. The phenomenological method of inquiry offers a way to gain insight into and examine these experiences so that they may be valued and shared with others in the community of nurses.

Paterson and Zderad insist that by sharing aspects of experiences with others, nurses confirm their own values and inspire others to value their experiences as well.

The valuing process translates into a reemphasis of the values and meanings central to each nurse's life world, a reassertion of the personal definition of the meaning of nursing, and, finally, personal and professional growth and satisfaction. Through this process, each nurse participates in keeping the idea of what it means to be a nurse in the forefront of consciousness.

Underpinning Paterson and Zderad's theory of humanistic nursing practice is a quasi-interpretive implementation of the phenomenological method of inquiry. Their method of implementation was specifically designed to teach nurses how to derive meanings from their nursing experiences, value those meanings, and share them with others. [Parts of the following are excerpted from Kleiman, 2005b.]

Paterson and Zderad describe five phases in their phenomenological study of nursing. Although these phases are presented in stepwise fashion, in actuality they are part of an intricately interrelated development of meaning. This dynamic may be thought of as a constant flow between, in all directions, and all-at-once emanating toward a center that is nursing. As presented by Paterson and Zderad, the phases of phenomenological inquiry are:

- Preparation of the nurse knower for coming to know
- Nurse knowing the other intuitively
- Nurse knowing the other scientifically
- Nurse complementarily synthesizing known others
- Succession within the nurse from the many to the paradoxical one

Preparation of the Nurse Knower for Coming to Know

In the first phase, the inquirer tries to open herself up to the unknown and possibly different. She consciously and conscientiously struggles with understanding and identifying her own angular view. The focus of an angular view is constrained by the field of vision of the observer. For example, if a nurse is looking at someone from the front she does not see what is in the back of the person. Instead the nurse makes instant assumptions based on previous experiences. For example, if the nurse sees red hair on a patient's head when she looks from the front, she assumes there is red hair on the back of the patient's head as well. Further, she assumes that the patient does, in fact, have a head in the back with hair on it.

There is also a perceptual angular view. Every nurse's internal visual field is clouded by, among other things, what may be thought of as her gestalt. A gestalt includes the inhered meanings and values that constitute the conceptual and experiential framework that individuals bring into any situation, a framework that is usually unexamined and casually accepted as we negotiate our everyday world. An individual's angular view is uniquely constituted by his gestalt and the perceptual and objective fields of reality that color the view at any given moment in time.

When engaging in the phenomenological method of inquiry, one must bracket his angular view in order to avoid distorting the meanings of the experiences being related. We must be aware that we have angular views derived from past and present experiences that are interpreted in the current moment. By being aware of our angular view and the dynamics of its qualities, we are then able to bracket it purposefully so that it is not superimposed on the meanings of the experiences we are trying to understand. We do not deny our unique selves, but we work to push our angular views into the background of discourse, allowing us to be open to the other's experience. This fundamental aspect of phenomenological inquiry helps us gain insight into that which the phenomenon reveals itself, in itself, to be. Later, the angular view is brought back into the foreground of consideration to help us make sense of, and give meaning to, the concrete experiences, their relevance for the phenomenon of interest and disciplinary perspectives, and as the validity of assumptions based on congruence with the data. Consider this description of the intended mindset of bracketing:

> I began to grasp the concept of bracketing a few years ago when I was traveling in Europe. As I visited each new country, I experienced the excitement of the unknown. I became aware of how alert, open, and other-directed I was in this uncharted world as compared with my daily routine at home. In my familiar surroundings, I would often fill in the blanks left by my inattentiveness to a routine experience, sometimes anticipating and answering questions even before they were asked.

This alertness, openness, and other-directedness is the goal of bracketing. Bracketing prepares the inquirer to enter the uncharted world of the other without expectations and preconceived ideas. It helps one to be open to the authentic, in other words, to the true experience of the other. Even temporarily letting go of that which shapes our own identity as the self, however, causes anxiety, fear, and uncertainty. Labeling, diagnosing, and routines add a necessary and very valuable predictability, sense of security, and means of conserving energy to our everyday existence and practice. Nevertheless, being open to the new and different is necessary for being able to know the other intuitively.

Nurse Knowing the Other Intuitively

Knowing the other intuitively is described by Paterson and Zderad as "moving back and forth between the impressions the nurse becomes aware of in herself and the recollected real experience of the other" (1976, pp. 88-89), which was obtained through the unbiased being with the other. The processes of bracketing and intuiting are not contradictory. Both are necessary and interwoven parts of the phenomenological process. The rigor and validity of phenomenology are based on continually referring back to the phenomenon itself. The process may be characterized as a dialectic between the impression and the real. Shifting back and forth allows for sudden insights on the part of the nurse, a new overall grasp that manifests itself in a clearer or perhaps a new "understanding." These understandings generate further development of the process. At this time, the nurse's general impressions are in a dialogue with her unbracketed view.

Nurse Knowing the Other Scientifically

Objectivity is needed as the nurse comes to know the other scientifically. Standing outside the phenomenon, the nurse examines it through analysis. She comes to know it through its parts or elements that are symbolic and known. This phase incorporates the nurse's ability to be conscious of herself and that which she has taken in, merged with, made part of herself. "This is the time when the nurse mulls over, analyzes, sorts out, compares, contrasts, relates, interprets, gives a name to, and categorizes" (Paterson & Zderad, 1976, p. 79).

For example, the nurse looks objectively at raw data such as temperature, blood pressure, and oxygen saturation; compares them to scientifically established medical parameters; draws upon her theoretical knowledge and practical experience in the natural and behavioral sciences; and analyzes the patient's status. These variances may also be related to developmental patterns or expected responses to trauma. This is when the nurse identifies deviations from norms and interprets and responds to degrees of variances.

Nurse Complementarily Synthesizing Known Others

At this point, the nurse personifies what has been described by Paterson and Zderad as a noetic locus, a knowing place (1976, p. 43). According to this concept, the greatest gift a human being can have is the ability to relate to others, to wonder, to search, to imagine about experience, and to create out of what has become known. Seeing themselves as "knowing places" inspires nurses to continue to develop and expand their community of world thinkers through their educational and practical experiences, which become a part of their angular view. This self-expansion, through the internalization of what others know, dynamically interrelates with the nurse's human capacity to be conscious of her own lived experiences. Through this interrelationship, the subjective and objective world of nursing can be reflected upon by each nurse, who is aware of and values herself as a "knowing place."

Succession Within the Nurse From the Many to the Paradoxical One

This is the birth of the new from the existing patterns, themes, and categories. It is in this phase that the nurse "comes up with a conception or abstraction that is inclusive of and beyond the multiplicities and contradictions" (Paterson & Zderad, 1976, p. 81) in a process that augments and expands her own angular view.

This is the dialectic process, which pervades every aspect of Humanistic Nursing Theory. In the dialectic process there is a repetitive pattern of organizing the dissimilar into a higher level (Barnum, 1990, p. 44) where differences are assimilated to create the new. The pervasive theme of dialectic assimilation speaks to universal interrelatedness, from the simplest to the most complex level. Human beings, by virtue of their ability to be self-observing, have the unique capacity to transcend themselves and reflect on their relationship to the universe. This dialectic may be observed in the call-and-response process described in Humanistic Nursing Theory. It describes the interactive dialogue between two human beings, from which a unique yet universal instance of nursing emerges. The nursing interaction is limited, but the internalization of that experience adds something new to each person's angular view. Neither person is the same as before. Each is more because of that coming together. The coming together of the nurse and the patient, the between in the lived world, is nursing. Just as in the double helix of the DNA molecule, this interweaving pattern is what structures the individual. In the fabric of Humanistic Nursing Theory this intentional interweaving between patient and nurse is what gives nursing its structure, form, and meaning. Box 6–2 contains an example of a study conducted using the phenomenological method in the style of Paterson and Zderad.

Phenomenology: Participating in a Community of Nurses

A report issued by the Secretary of Health and Human Services' Commission on Nursing in December 1988 stated, "The perspective and expertise of nurses are a

Box 6–2 | Oliveira, Nailze Figueiredo Souza. *Lived dialogue between nurse and mothers of children with cancer,* **2003. 107f. Dissertation (Master's Degree)—Centro de Ciências da Saúde/Universidade Federal da Paraíba, João Pessoa.**

The gradual increase of the number of cases of children with cancer on the Brazilian scene has alarmed many health professionals responsible for research into quality care for this clientele and their families. In health units directed toward the treatment of childhood cancer, it is clearly observed that the mother and/or relative most frequently accompany the child, whether for ambulatory treatment or hospitalization. Thus, the person accompanying the child becomes a client who needs nursing care as well. This study consists of field research of a qualitative nature, with the objective of understanding the lived dialogue between nurses and mothers of children with cancer, illuminated by Paterson and Zderad's Theory of Humanistic Nursing. The participants of the study were six mothers who accompanied their children with cancer in the Pediatrics Unit of Hospital Napoleão Laureano, which serves cancer clients in the city of João Pessoa, Paraiba, in the period from October through December, 2002. The lived dialogue was developed on the basis of the phases of Phenomenological Nursing. The first phase—preparation of the nurse to come to know—consisted of seeking self-knowledge as prerequisite to come to know mothers of children with cancer. In the second phase—the nurse knows the other intuitively—arose encounters with the mothers in the pediatric unit, moments in which there were calls and responses of an I-Thou nature. In this phase, the data emerged from the encounters between nurse and mothers through the interview technique and were recorded in a field diary. The rest of the phases served as the basis for analysis of data, constituting the moments of the I-Thou relation: the nurse knows the other scientifically; the nurse synthesized in a way in which known realities and the multiple realities became a paradoxical unity. The following categories emerged from data analysis: the mothers before the discovery of the diagnosis; mothers before treatment of the child; mothers before adaptation to the hospital environment; mothers lacking information; mothers with problems in the context of family; mothers whose physical health and emotions were affected; mothers searching for ways of facing up to the situation; mothers living moments of joy. The lived dialogue, intuitively and scientifically, made it possible for the mothers to receive care that promoted their well being and more being in the lived experience.

necessary adjunct to that of other health care professionals in the policy-making, and regulatory, and standard setting process" (p. 31). This mandate is still echoed in today's nursing literature (Wick, 2003), confirming the belief that nurses are still challenged to help bring about change in the health-care system.

In response to this challenge, a group of nurses joined together to help actualize the power of the profession. The result is a phenomenological reflection on nurses' experiences struggling with change in the nursing role. The researcher reflected on her own experiences as a nurse manager struggling with changes happening around and affecting her. Normally, in settings such as hospitals, the time pressures, the unending tasks, and the emotional strains and conflicts do not allow nurses to relate, reflect, and support each other in their struggle toward a center that is nursing. The result is isolation and alienation that do not allow for the development of either a personal or professional voice.

Within the community of nurses, it became clear that developing individual voices was the first task. Talking and listening to each other about their nursing worlds allowed them to become more articulate and clear about function and value as nurses. The theme of developing an articulate voice pervaded and continues to pervade this group. There is an ever-increasing awareness of both manner and language as the group members interact among themselves and with those outside of the group. The resolve for an articulate voice is even more firm as members of the group experience and share the empowering effect it can have on their personal and professional lives. It has been said that "those that express themselves unfold in health, beauty, and human potential. They become unblocked channels through which creativity can flow" (Hills & Stone, 1976, p. 71).

Group members offered alternative approaches to various situations. For example, nurses shared experiences where their input was marginalized; they offered ways to present their points of view in a confident and assertive manner. At times role-playing was used to refine approaches and get feedback. This process also helped group members to explore strategies to deal with the increasing responsibilities of leadership and the challenge of instituting change. Members were supported when they had negative experiences, and when a particular approach worked nurses shared it with others. In this way, each member's experience became available to all members as members individually formulated their own knowledge base and expanded their angular view, thereby becoming more of a "knowing place" within the community of nurses.

Through openness and sharing, the group members were able to differentiate their strengths. Once they could truly appreciate the unique competence of the other, the group members were able to reflect that appreciation back. Through reflection, members began to learn that positive mirroring did not have to come from outsiders. Internalizing and then projecting a competent image reflects back on the other an image of competence and power.

As a community, nurses can empower each other. This reciprocity is a self-enhancing process, for "the degree to which I can create relationships which facilitate the growth of others as separate persons is a measure of the growth I have achieved in myself" (Rogers, 1976, p. 79). Thus, by sharing in our community of nurses, we can empower each other through mutual confirmation as we help each other move toward a center that is nursing.

REFERENCES

Alford, R. (1998). *The craft of inquiry: Theories, methods, evidence.* New York: Oxford University Press.

Barnum, B. (1990). *Nursing theory: Analysis, application, evaluation.* Glenview, Ill.: Scott, Foresman/Little, Brown.

Giorgi, A. (1997). The theory, practice, and evaluation of the phenomenological method as a qualitative research procedure. *Journal of Phenomenological Psychology*, 28(2), 235.

Giorgi, A. (2003). *The philosophy and methodology of phenomenological inquiry.* Workshop given at University of Quebec, Montreal, Canada.

Hills, C., & Stone, R. B. (1976). *Conduct your own awareness sessions: 100 ways to enhance self-concept in the classroom.* Englewood Cliffs, N.J.: Prentice-Hall.

Husserl, E, (1913/1972). *Ideas: General introduction to pure phenomenology*, trans. W.R. Boyce. Gibson, N.Y.: Collier.

Kleiman, S. (2004a). What is the nature of nurse practitioners' lived-experiences interacting with patients? *Journal of the American Academy of Nurse Practitioners*, 16(6), 263–269.

Kleiman, S. (2004b). Phenomenology: To wonder and search for meaning. *Nurse Researcher*, 11(4), 7–19.

Kleiman, S. (2005b). Josephine Paterson and Loretta Zderad's humanistic nursing theory and its applications. In M. Parker (Ed.), *Nursing theories and nursing practice* (2nd ed., pp. 125-137). Philadelphia: F.A. Davis.

Merleau-Ponty, M. (1962). *Phenomenology of perception,* trans. C. Smith. 1958. New York: Routledge & Kegan Paul.

Oliveira, N. (2003). Lived dialogue between nurse and mothers of children with cancer. 107f. Dissertation (master's degree)—Centro de Ciências da Saúde/ Universidade Federal da Paraíba, João Pessoa.

Palmer, R. (1999). *Hermeneutics and the disciplines.* Lecture delivered at the Department of Philosophy, Southern Illinois University at Carbondale. Retrieved March 1, 2003, from http://www.mac.edu/~rpalmer/

Parse, R. (2003). The lived-experience of feeling very tired: A study using the Parse research method. *Nursing Science Quarterly* 16(4), 319–325.

Paterson, J., & Zderad, L. (1976). *Humanistic nursing.* New York: Wiley.

Rogers, C. (1976). *Perceiving, behaving, and becoming: 100 ways to enhance self concept in the classroom.* Englewood Cliffs, NJ: Prentice-Hall.

Schutz, A. (1970). *On phenomenology and social relations: Selected writings.* Chicago: Chicago University of Chicago Press.

U.S. Public Health Services. (12/88). *Secretary's commission on nursing, final report.* Washington, DC: Department of Health & Human Services.

Wick, G. (2003). A place where the spirit can grow: An answer to recruitment and retention? *Nephrology Nursing Journal.* 30(1).

Wyatt, C. (2003). Existentialism and Jean-Paul Sartre. Retrieved April 20, 2003, from http://www.tameri.com/csw/exist/sartre.asp#quotes

Permissions

Excerpts from the following publications were used in this chapter:

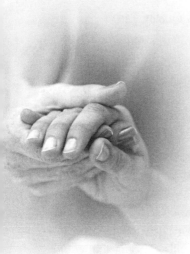

Chapter 7

Culture as a Component of Human Centered Nursing

In a highly diverse environment, a nurse cannot anticipate what kind of specific cultural knowledge will be necessary to serve her next patient. She does not have time to research or study about cultural attributes for a future or even present patient. However, approaching a particular patient with assumptions about his cultural affinities is impertinent. Presumed familiarity can have just as negative an effect on the relationships formed with patients and families (Schutz, 1944) as can disregard for cultural characteristics.

As part of their practice as health-care providers, nurses must be sensitive to culturally inhered meanings that individuals possess. Such sensitivity facilitates the delivery of quality care and has the potential to enhance patient outcomes (U.S. Department of Health and Human Services, 2000; Leininger, 2001).

What Is Culture and Why Is It a Relevant Aspect of Human Centered Nursing?

Insight into the origin and genesis of the idea of culture as an aspect of human affairs is provided by "The Allegory of the Well." This fable was inspired, in part, by the works on culture and language of Levi-Strauss (1983) and Rousseau (1966).

> Once upon a time in pre-history when humankind (human beings) first inhabited the earth, they presented with certain requirements for the sustenance of life. These included the naturally occurring elements of air to breathe and water to drink or quench thirst. Also necessary was food to eat or dispel hunger and maintain biological stability. Food occurred in nature as meat or fowl from animals, vegetation from plants and trees, and fish from the waters of the sea or lakes and streams. These were probably eaten raw or putrefied in the very beginning

before the discovery of fire and other preparation techniques for alter-ing palatability and digestibility. Because of the simple need to survive, human beings were drawn to areas of dwelling where this sustenance was, if not plentiful, at least available.

Because the surface of the planet was already enveloped in air, the first priority in choosing an area in which to dwell was its proximity to water to drink—a well. Not everyone could live very near to the well, drinking and bathing at will, so persons would travel to the well, retrieve water in some kind of receptacle, and carry it back to the place of abode for future use. Because water is heavy, the amount that could be carried was limited by the strength of the carrier or carriers and the distance to and from the well. Frequent trips were necessary. Along the way and during the time spent at the well one would encounter other people and animals that inhabited a given area. By the way others pre-sented themselves—moving, breathing, walking, making sounds, threat-ening, keeping distance—people were able to recognize others who appeared to be similar in nature to themselves.

Mental images of others would be formed based on their size, stature, sex, speed and efficiency with which they practiced their tasks, for example. Also telling were details about whether they traveled alone or in groups, and the extent to and manner in which they exchanged some form of recognition or greeting. Recognition would evoke curios-ity, and except in the case of perceived danger, would engender attempts to interact or at least communicate.

As people confronted each other more and more frequently, they developed a protocol or social practice for introduction and/or recognition—of waving or nodding or even responding to cries of pain, sorrow, distress, or joy. This was probably manifested in certain sounds a person might make when approaching or recognizing another and that person mimicking the same sound in affirming some form of meaning. One possibility may be a shout of warning when a dangerous animal or hostile human being was approaching. Others may include a child crying out in pain after injuring himself while playing, a person smiling after quenching thirst or recognizing another who evoked some unexplained sensation of pleasure.

As the visits to the well became more frequent and other types of encounters happened (hunting or fleeing from animals, gathering or meeting along the way) more and more protocols and linguistic forms evolved. As the encounters became more frequent and the social inter- actions between people became more extensive and complex, a whole array of sounds were [sic] born and used by people trying to express their feelings or meanings for a situation to another or others. Humans, as beings with the unique ability to "think," quickly recognized the use- fulness of these sounds for the purpose of conveying thoughts and emotions as opposed to the tedious process of "showing" another "how to" as a mode of communication. This phenomenon offers us insight into the origin and development of language as a medium through which we can express both our historical and current con- sciousness and as a mode of understanding each other (Gadamer, 1989, pp. xxxiv–xxxv).

Of course, the Allegory of the Well is just that, as there are no verifiable recordings of these happenings. They are, however, contrivances of imagination that are based on observations of people's responses to events, which add to specu- lation on the evolution of social structures, language, and culture.

The World as We Know It

From these crude beginnings of civilization, the world as we know it can be extrapo- lated. Behaviors evolved over centuries into social constructions of the way certain people interact with people of the same persuasion as well as with those of different persuasions. For example, the way peoples celebrated certain rites of passage, infancy, adolescence, marriage, childbirth, courtesy protocols, etc., were taught and carried for- ward from generation to generation. These rites received little scrutiny or challenge.

As the problems of distance between peoples were overcome, groups adopted the practice of identifying themselves as well as other groups by the way they appeared in public. Each group compared the way it conducted itself in public and private discourse and action with the appearance and behaviors of other groups. The sum of the qualities of similar individuals and groups is called "culture," and the way groups manifest their culture is "their mode of social interaction." Language, too, is a mode of social interaction, and a very economical one, through which many aspects of culture and the meanings associated with it are defined and conveyed (Gadamer, 1989, pp. xxxv–xxxvi). One way language is used to convey aspects of culture in health care and nursing is by communicating information about desires and limitations on treatments. For example, culture comes through in patients' perspectives on blood transfusions, birth and dying, designation of advocates, special needs, and understanding of their rights as patients.

Some of the modes of interaction common to a group or subgroup came to be required or mandated as part of consideration for entry into or retention of membership in the group. That is, members of a particular group or subgroup believe certain behaviors are the "right" or morally correct way to behave in a given situation. When these so-called morally correct behaviors become widely accepted, required, or mandated, they are called laws, rules, or ethics. The subject of ethics as it applies to nursing or human centered nursing will be discussed in the next chapter.

The process of developing cultures has evolved over thousands of years and is still evolving. In fact, modes of transportation and communication are developing at such an accelerated pace that they profoundly influence culture, cultural awareness, cultural sensitivity, and cultural competence, all necessary components of being with patients. This is because of the resulting virtual closeness of many people in the world. For example, people in the Western world can turn a switch and observe peoples of many different cultures or pick up the telephone—the first virtual reality instrument—and within seconds talk to someone anywhere in the world.

Furthermore, while walking down the street in a large metropolitan area, one is apt to pass tens or hundreds of different peoples and their emblems of their cultural heritage: attire, music, cuisine, and ceremony. Of course, the denser and more diverse the population a nurse serves, the more acute the issue of cultural sensitivity is. Cultural mixing complicates matters because as cultures commingle, some members of groups find the behaviors, mannerisms, and attributes of a neighboring culture appealing and adopt them as their own either as a process of augmentation or replacement. Alternately, people may find some of the attributes of a particular group so distasteful that they discredit any individual believed to be part of that group. It follows that nurses can expect that the persons they serve may have a wide variety of cultural attributes and perceptions of the world different from their own. This phenomenon is amplified because, among the nursing population, there are nurses who serve diverse communities and who have themselves diverse cultural backgrounds. Furthermore, and perhaps most important to this discussion, because of the intimacy of the relationship between nurses and patients, the cultural affinities of each affect and effect the type of service to be provided and accepted.

Of lesser intimacy, but still of importance, is respect for cultural disposition between student and teacher. For example, at one time in one institution, 16 different countries of origin were represented in one class of 25 students. Each class consisted of a diverse population of students from many countries having varied and interesting cultural backgrounds. In the neighborhood where the school was located and students had clinical placements, 115 languages were spoken by people from 145 countries. This type of population distribution presents unparalleled opportunities for the teacher to role-model and demonstrate cultural competence as well as for students to study culture and its importance in nurse/patient relationships.

The key questions present in the area of cultural practice include:

- How does a nurse acquire cultural awareness?
- How does a nurse acquire cultural sensitivity?
- How does a nurse become culturally competent?
- How are nursing students prepared to thrive in this complex milieu?

A mode of inquiry into cultural sensitivity is needed to give nurses a spontaneous action template for any person of any culture, a practical mode of being with patients and families that complements their cultural differences despite the inherent difficulties of such a project. A good starting point for this endeavor is establishing some working definitions applicable to the study of culture in human centered nursing.

Culture

In its broadest sense, culture may be defined as the totality of socially transmitted behavior patterns, arts, beliefs, institutions, predominating attitudes, and other products of human work and thought that characterize the functioning of a group (Bodley, 1994). All the characteristics of the everyday life of a people represent the whole of its culture and become markers by which cultural assignments are made. These include learned behaviors, social organization, language, values, and beliefs that are the expression of a particular group or subgroup. Culture can also refer to social class or membership in a special population; for example, middle class, privileged, mentally ill, disabled, teenager, or elderly.

Cultural Awareness, Sensitivity, and Competence

Cultural awareness, cultural sensitivity, and cultural competence are not new concerns for nursing practice and nursing education. It has been argued for at least 45 years that knowledge of patients' cultural attributes affects the quality of nursing care (Leininger, 2001). Recognition of and responsiveness to cultural differences are considered central to providing quality care (Heller, et al., 2000; Leininger, 2001; Ludwig, & Silva, 2000). Moreover, the failure to recognize a patient's culture and customs can have a negative impact on patients (U.S. Department of Health and Human Services, 2000). For example, the child brought to a nurse practitioner complaining of stomach pain and thirst may be wrongly diagnosed as diabetic if the nurse is unaware that certain foods are commonly eaten by persons of the child's ethnic background (Leininger, 2001).

The terms *cultural awareness, cultural sensitivity*, and *cultural competence* are used frequently in the literature. For the purposes of this chapter, they are defined as follows:

- Cultural awareness is a learned or epiphenomenally acquired awareness that diverse peoples live and thrive within some cultural context, both inherited and experiential, that is particular to their group.

- Cultural sensitivity is the belief that attention to cultural contexts within which patients thrive promotes beneficial outcomes in nursing care and influences what care will be provided, how that care will be provided, and what care may or may not be accepted by patients and families.

- Cultural competence, which encompasses cultural awareness and cultural sensitivity, includes immediate and acquired knowledge about an individual's cultural affinities and the skills and willingness to integrate these cultural affinities into the delivery of nursing care.

Bringing Culture Into the Classroom and Clinic

In the classroom setting, students are taught to look for and recognize cultural issues important to patients and families. They are urged to integrate aspects of cultural awareness, cultural sensitivity, and cultural competence consistent with the recognition of each individual as a unique personality. The approach generally integrates the theoretical precepts of Leininger's comparative cultural caring model (Leininger, 2001) and Paterson and Zderad's humanistic nursing model (1976). These theoretical groundings are actualized through the activities of the Humanistic Teaching Model relevant to the study of culture and integrated into the clinical setting. An example of this integration is represented by the following incident:

After reviewing her assigned patient's chart, she entered the patient's room and introduced herself as a nursing student in keeping with the approach discussed in pre-conference. The patient responded by asking, 'Are you an Egyptian?' Flustered and disarmed by this unanticipated response, the student excused herself and sought her instructor.

The student spoke to the instructor about her impulse to flee the room and her fear that the patient was rejecting her because of an apparent identification with September 11, 2001, terrorists. The instructor helped the student identify that her experience of being objectified by a cultural classification had an emotional impact on her that interfered with her ability to engage in an intersubjective interaction with her patient. In this situation, the student did not understand what the remark implied for the patient.

With support, the nursing student reflected on the experience and understood the need to approach the patient again in an attempt to gain an understanding of what the patient meant by the remark. As it turned out, the patient had identified something in the student's appearance that reminded him of the friendly people he had known when he had traveled to Egypt many years before. The student came to understand that the patient's cultural identification of her was an attempt to know something about her and relate to her.

This experience helped the nursing student understand how a person's positive intentions can lead to negative results when a cultural classification proceeds under false assumptions. Classification to a group as the only means of relating to a person negates the uniqueness of each individual and can alienate rather than foster an "I-and-thou" relationship.

Comparative Cultural Caring Model

Leininger's model, based on ethnographic studies, requires that nurses be competent in caring for patients from more than one culture. She argues that individuals have attributes that can be aligned with cultural profiles and that nurses can provide care consistent with that alignment. She gathered a catalog of approximately 100 cultures, with their associated attributes from ethnographic studies (Leininger, 2001).

The main advantage of this approach is that nurses completely unfamiliar with cultures other than their own, a form of ethnocentrism, would have some documented evidence available to them that raises their awareness of the fact that there are diverse peoples that have lifeways consistent with groups other than their own. In general, ethnocentrism refers to an explicit or implicit assumption of one's own culture as being superior to that of others. Ethnocentrism may also entail a total lack of awareness that another culture even exists. See Box 7–1.

Box 7–1 | Ethnocentrism

An example of ethnocentrism as a complicating factor in achieving cultural competence and how it is applicable to nursing is given in the following adventure of a group of World Bank managers in Sri Lanka. One of the engineers relates the story:

In order to improve the cultural competence of a group of World Bank managers, we sent them to live in villages for 2 weeks and experience, among other things, poverty first hand. So we went with about 10 people and [...]stayed in a village called Wampalesa. The home in which we spent the night had a single family head. The husband was out in the north part of Sri Lanka because of the civil conflict, leaving three children behind with their mother, who was raising the children on her own.

In the evening we all needed to take a bath so we asked where we could go. Obviously there was no tap inside, so we walked and found a very large pond of water, which was the only source of water for the village. So we go in, because you had to find some way to get cleaned up from the dust and so on, and just as we put our feet in everyone started shouting that we should leave because the elephants were coming. That water source was not only for drinking water, but also for bathing and all hygiene needs, as well as a watering source for the elephants. [...] The water source was the central gathering place where everything and everyone intersected, as well as the place where these diverse and primitive peoples developed some of the attributes and qualities of their life-ways. In order to understand and relate to peoples different from ourselves,[...] it is important for us to learn how to take opportunities for improving cultural competence in diverse settings as a dynamic event.

From this adventure we can also learn that although we set out on a task with the very best of intentions ready to demonstrate our acumen in solving problems—bringing to bear all the latest technological wonders and techniques at our disposal—it is awareness and sensitivity to the demeanor and life-ways of the people involved that is the most important aspect of our mode of delivering services. And it is this sensitivity that has a lot to do with the perception of the success or failure of our project insofar as our clients are concerned (MIT Leadership Center, 2006).

The story in Box 7–1 has several lessons for health care and, in particular, human centered nursing. First, it is essential to recognize that patients and families may have backgrounds and life-ways entirely different from those in the West. For example, the engineers in the story imagined the noble goal of bringing running water into every household. The people of the village, however, said that they would be satisfied with just some kind of damming or pooling of the water so that they could use it separate from the elephants and other animals. This would be a smaller project, requiring less time and money, and would satisfy the modest needs of the natives.

Modern health care often launches into a heroic effort against sickness and injury, bringing to bear the latest technology and procedures—chemotherapy, radiation therapy, organ transplantation, artificial life extension—making assumptions about what is and is not consistent with patients' and families' basic values and meanings for life. But in this determination to serve patients, the individuality and dignity of those served are not respected; in other words, they are not served in a culturally competent manner. In terms of the precepts of human centered nursing, this entails remembering that people interact with people, not with a disease, and ask, "What is it that the patient wants and considers to be quality care?"

Furthermore, being culturally competent is more complex and difficult than merely recognizing and accommodating "differences," even if one could possibly catalog all the cultures of the world. Schutz (1944) pointed out some of the deficiencies in using the cataloging or classification approach. He cautions against one person raised in one culture coming into the culture of another with a fixed notion of the community she is entering.

In particular, when a nurse assumes the role of an observer and tries objectively to reconstruct the patient's rules for the patient's practical conduct for everyday life according to some ethnographer's catalog of cultural norms, the nurse's position becomes one of un-involvement. Even if the nurse accepts the patient's routine behavior, it will be perceived as being void of an understanding of the underlying spirit of the native community. In both instances the nurse remains an outsider to the patient and the patient's experiences.

What this means is that an attitude of familiarity with some culturally binding attributes of a particular culture does not necessarily give one entry into that community, nor does it lead to acceptance and trust by patients or their relatives. An "objective" cultural view of the patient may lead the nurse to act erroneously in what she believes to be a culturally competent manner toward the patient. But being an objective observer and "student" of a particular culture does not necessarily lead to an understanding of the patient's individual acculturation. This is an important point because familiarity can backfire. The nurse's presumed familiarity with a patient's culture and beliefs may be interpreted as offensive and disrespectful, thus distancing the nurse from the patient and hindering, rather than helping, the implementation of the care plan. The main disadvantage of this approach is that the lived experiences or existential quality of personal experiences are sacrificed for the cultural, social, or global focus. That is, the more difficult task of looking for individuality in a patient is set aside in favor of categorizing the patient according to some class or type of personality.

Humanistic Nursing (Intersubjective Relationship) Model

Paterson and Zderad's model emphasizes the uniqueness of individuals and stresses the primacy of understanding the subjective meanings each individual assigns to a situation, regardless of his apparent, or not so apparent, ethnic or cultural appearances and characteristics. Characterized by open and attentive attitudes toward patients and their health-care needs, the intersubjective approach is free of presuppositions or judgments. Patients are viewed as unique human beings with their own sets of subjective meanings that they assign to their life situations. These include culturally inhered meanings, as well as other influences, such as social behaviors, historical and environmental phenomena, and aspirations for the future—all of which may have an effect on their perceptions of their health-related needs and the treatments they anticipate and will or will not accept.

This personally directed approach is supported by the belief that a prerequisite to quality nursing care is the intersubjective relationship between the nurse and patient (Benner & Wrubel, 1989; Forchuk, 1991; Henderson, 1964; Paterson & Zderad, 1976; Watson, 1999). Of course, one might argue that this approach characterizes what nurses have always done and that it represents nothing new. But in light of a perception of technology as a replacement for the nursing act, e.g., computer monitoring of patient's vital signs, nursing is challenged to remain vital and relevant to the patient as person.

Humanistic Teaching Model

As with all aspects of the Humanistic Nursing Theory as outlined in this book, a series of exercises are used to lead students through both the theoretical and practical applications of cultural awareness, cultural sensitivity, and cultural competence so they can be integrated into nursing practice.

Exercise 1 directs attention to Leininger's Comparative Cultural Caring Model, its structure and some of its benefits and limitations. The question is: "To what extent would a student know a culture by virtue of setting down attributes of persons belonging to that culture, and to what extent are these attributes useful in students' extrapolation to patient experiences?" Exercise 2 directs attention to the intersubjective perspective by involving students in one-to-one interactions with classmates and patients. This familiarizes them with the possibilities of individual nuance within a cultural context.

Exercise 1

This exercise, following from Leininger's Comparative Cultural Caring Model, has two purposes: (1) to make students aware that, regardless of one's cultural affiliation, one may or may not have specific observable values, beliefs, and traditions grounded in one's cultural affinities; and (2) to teach students that skill and proficiency in understanding and implementing cultural preferences have a positive impact on the quality of nursing care.

Activities. Students are asked to identify their cultural affiliation and are divided into groups according to their affiliation. Students experience the difficulty of finding a precise cultural group and puzzle over the various differences engendered by place of birth, where they were raised, and the environmental considerations that affect how one determines what one's culture is. For example, a student of Indian descent raised in the Caribbean who has adopted Caribbean behaviors may identify with the Caribbean culture rather than the Indian culture. Each group prepares a presentation on the characteristics of the group, including such aspects as values, traditions, ethnicity, beliefs, food, and attire.

Expected Outcomes. As students learn that there are differences even among people of the same cultural backgrounds, they will become aware that people appreciate recognition of their cultural assignments. They will also recognize that some of the assumptions they have had about their own culture and the cultures of others in the class are incorrect.

Observed Outcomes. Students are averse to both self-classification and to being classified by others. Although they reject classification that entails prejudgment with respect to their beliefs and values, they do not reject their own cultural attributes and report being proud of them.

- Students learn that belonging to a cultural group does not necessarily predict responses to situational contexts or individual needs but can provide clues that help in understanding the person.

- Students become aware of the need for tolerance of similarities and differences with regard to their relationships with patients. For example, one student reports being told that many Hispanic women in the maternity ward hold their babies in a certain way to avoid the "evil eye" or "mal ojo" (a belief that excessive praise or showing too much attention to the child results in harm). Another student, noting the importance of spirituality in each culture, regardless of the practices or rituals that are performed, states, "Spiritual beliefs of a patient should be respected regardless of their differences from my own beliefs."

- Being exposed to and confronted with different cultures and observing the way people of these cultures approach situations are acknowledged as important lessons for nursing students. Students assume open-mindedness to the possibilities of other ways of looking at and being present with their patients.

- Students learn that patients need to be encountered as individuals who may or may not conform to the norms of the culture to which they belong, and they learn to encounter each patient freshly, to avoid typecasting the patient according to preconceived ideas.

The group presentations highlight a number of markers characteristic of the cultures represented, including music, cuisine, and folk medicine, healers, and treatment modalities.

- Music, including differences in rhythms, tonalities, and instruments, is observed to be a consistent cultural marker used by the different groups. For example, the fact that some cultures play and sing high-spirited music at funerals and others play somber music may give clues to how groups view death and dying.

- Similarities in cuisine are associated with various cultural groups. For example, the meat pies eaten in South America, India, and Jamaica are quite similar in appearance and taste, and people from Africa, the Philippines, and Latino cultures all favor rice and beans.

Differences are noted as well. For example, the fact that some cultures do not eat meat products from certain animals, or avoid meat or dairy products altogether, may have a religious significance. The importance of the family gathering at meals has social significance in many cultures.

- Faith in folk medicines, healers, and treatments for certain illnesses is a distinguishing feature woven through the presentations. Many African, Caribbean, and South American cultures are amenable to medicines that are unfamiliar to health-care professionals in Western society, and some cultures believe that voodoo holds power over an individual's health.

Exercise 2

The purpose is to have students learn the techniques and efficacy of the intersubjective approach by engaging in one-on-one interaction and dialogue about their personal interpretations of their particular culture.

Activities. Students are divided into pairs representing two different cultural heritages. Within each pair, students discuss values, beliefs, and experiences in an effort to recognize and understand the meanings assigned to them by persons culturally different from themselves. Later, students share what they have learned and their reactions to engaging in the exercise with the other students in the class. A dialogue between two students becomes an open discussion among all students. Other students from the culture being discussed are especially active in contributing their own knowledge, perceptions, and experiences.

Expected Outcomes. Students become aware of their own cultural beliefs and values, have the opportunity to explore a different culture from a subjective point of view, and develop an open attitude toward other cultures by gaining insight into their preconceived ideas.

Observed Outcomes. Students report learning about cultural attitudes toward family, religion, food, education, social mobility, rituals, gender roles, language, and health-care beliefs by sharing insights into their own beliefs and examining similarities and differences between and within cultures. They learn the value of integrating cultural issues into patient interactions.

Examples of student comments related to this exercise follow. The following list relates to Asian cultures.

- "Men are decision makers, and I should know who in the family makes the decisions."
- "I need to be aware of gestures that have a lot of meaning to persons from this culture."
- "I learned that in some Asian cultures pain is expressed in various ways. Language often poses a barrier. If they are in pain, they may not verbalize it because they feel that they are not understood."
- "The family system is more rigid, and they keep family issues to themselves. The nurse needs to restrict her commentary to health-related issues and how they will affect the person and his life."
- "They believe that family members or friends staying with the ill person is very important."

Dialogues within the student pairs and discussion among the class members pointed to differences and similarities between and within cultures:

- "Our cultures sort of mirror each other, having similar values and beliefs, except expressing them in different ways."
- "I found out that even though we have different cultures, different ethnicity, we have similar values and beliefs, such as we don't express emotional feelings in public, our need for privacy when grieving, men are the head of the household."
- "I experience that my culture, Hispanic, is in some ways similar to his African culture. For example, they respect the elderly and nature. We also respect the elderly. I experienced a sense of getting new knowledge from a culture rich in traditions, like their strong love for nature and respect for the elderly. I learned that we share almost the same values, but they don't show emotions in relation to a dead person. My preconceived idea was that they would have to show their emotions when somebody dies, because my culture is very expressive, they faint and they cry a lot."

The students also became aware that although there may be similarities between cultures, individuals within a culture are unique.

- "I realized that I'm not bounded by culture, so my experiences, beliefs, and values may be different from every Jamaican in this class."

- "I learned that even though individuals might be from the same country, we couldn't presuppose that their values, beliefs, and culture are the same."

- "Nigerians have different beliefs and values. This is dependent on the village they are from. My preconceived idea was that all Nigerians had the same values and beliefs and were from the same culture, but now I know that's not true."

Remarks from students reflected an increasing awareness of the complexity of the individual and the various influences beyond cultural background that have an affect on individuals.

- "I learned that I might not be as aware of my culture as I thought because I grew up with my family at home and they're my point of reference. My beliefs might not be similar to the culture as a whole."

- "I learned that although we are different ages and come from different places, many of the experiences upon coming into the American culture were very similar in terms of how we view certain things that are maybe less acceptable to our original culture. I learned that my beliefs and values are more to the American culture versus my original culture, but perhaps that's due to social and economic status."

Through the exercises, students learn to be alert to culturally binding attributes of individual patients. They learn that knowledge about various cultures provides clues to how individuals may react but that each patient, regardless of her cultural affiliation, is a unique individual involved in a direct, intersubjective interaction with her nurse and must be acknowledged as such. In the final analysis, students learn that attention to culturally inherent meanings as they apply to particular individuals, contributes to beneficial outcomes in nursing care.

REFERENCES

Benner, P., & Wrubel, J. (1989). *The primacy of caring.* New York: Addison Wesley.

Bodley, J. (1994). *Cultural anthropology: Tribes, states, and the global system.* Mountain View, Calif.: Mayfield.

Forchuk, C. (1991). Peplau's theory: Concepts and their relations. *Nursing Science Quarterly,* 4(2), 54–60.

Gadamer, H. (1989). *Truth and method. Second revised edition*, trans. Joel Weinsheimer and Donald G. Marshall. New York: Continuum International.

Heller, B. R., Oros, M. T., & Durney-Crowley, J. (2000). The future of nursing education: Ten trends to watch. *Nursing and Health Care Perspectives*, 21, 9–13.

Henderson, V. (1964). The nature of nursing. *American Journal of Nursing*, 64(8), 62–67.

Leininger, M. (2001). A mini-journey into transcultural nursing with its founder. *Nebraska Nurse*, 34, 2, 16–23.

Levi-Strauss. (1983). *The Raw and the cooked*, translated John and Doreen Weightman. University of Chicago Press.

Ludwig, R., & Silva, M. C. (2000). Nursing around the world: Cultural values and ethical conflicts. *Online Journal of Issues in Nursing*. Available at http://www.nursingworld.org/ojin/ethicol/ethics_4.htm

MIT Leadership Center. (2006). Leading across boundaries. Accessed April 4, 2006, from http://mitworld.mit.edu/video/307/

Paterson, J., & Zderad, L. T. (1976). *Humanistic nursing*. New York: Wiley.

Rousseau, J. (1966). *Essay on the origin of language*, trans., with afterword, John H. Moran and Alexander Code. University of Chicago Press.

Schutz, A. (1944). The stranger: An essay in social psychology. *American Journal of Sociology*, 49, 499–507.

U.S. Department of Health and Human Services. (2000). *Healthy people 2010: Understanding and improving health*, 2nd ed. Washington, DC: U.S. Government Printing Office.

Watson, J. (1999). *Postmodern nursing and beyond*. Edinburgh, Scotland: Churchill Livingstone/WB Saunders.

Permissions

Excerpts from:

Kleiman, S., Frederickson, K., & Lundy, T. (2004). Using an eclectic model to educate students about cultural influences on the nurse-patient relationship. *Nursing Education Perspectives* 25(5), 249–253.

Used by permission of the National League for Nursing

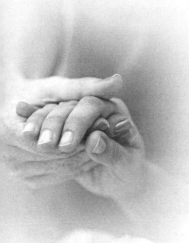

Chapter 8

Ethics and Human Centered Nursing

Many activities, behaviors, and interactions in civilized society are scrutinized, commented upon, and judged within the various constituents of ethically accepted and mandated guidelines. The concern about ethics in nursing, and particularly human centered nursing, derives from the fact that nursing requires interactions and interrelationships between and among people.

The origin of many of ethical priorities evolved from the idea of culture. Culture was defined as an evolving process through which certain behaviors of members of groups become required or mandated as criteria for inclusion or retention in a group or sub-group (see Chapter 7). Over time some of these behaviors are raised to the level of being "morally correct"; that is, connoting or denoting good or bad or right or wrong as regards individuals or the community. When the so-called morally correct behaviors become widely accepted, required, or mandated—and insofar as they point to a body or set of principles for right conduct—they are called rules, laws, or ethics. These are often codified and recorded in some form of writing and generally accepted as authoritative for a designated population.

In the professional community of nursing there are rules, laws, a code of ethics, and other guidelines that nurses need to be familiar with and ultimately rely on to guide their practice. Rather than deferring or referring to authority figures outside the profession, nurses need to rely on their own knowledge of their professional and legal responsibilities and be competent in accessing authoritative professional documents to inform and support themselves. Nurses also need to be familiar with their professional organizations as resources.

Rules, Laws, and Ethics

It is important first to distinguish between the various levels of behavioral mandate.

Rules

Rules may be defined as common practice guides for behaviors, e.g., getting in line in crowded situations, promptness, times of starting and ending a shift, appropriate dress, manner of salutation, and other mundane events. Rules do not necessarily have a moral basis, but they may, as in the case of respectful courtesy protocols in addressing one's elders, juniors, companions, and dignitaries.

Laws

Laws are the binding principles of government that are constructed and recorded by legislative bodies. Laws focus on the welfare and interest of the general population and, for the most part, have their bases in morality and justice. They are interpreted by the court system of judges and enforced under penalties said to be consistent with the sensitivity of the community. In nursing, legal obligations to the public are defined in the nurse practice acts. Each state and territory of the United States has a form of nurse practice act, available on the Internet, that defines the scope of practice and responsibilities of nurses at all levels of practice. These statutes are used in legal proceedings to adjudicate infractions, noncompliance, liability, and other matters. Every nurse and student nurse needs to be familiar with the state practice act. It is the legal responsibility of all nurses to know what they are licensed to do and to know what is outside their scope of practice.

Nurse Practice Acts

Every state and territory has a nurse practice act that defines the scope of nursing practice and is overseen by boards of nursing. In addition, nurse practice acts mandate requirements for entry into nursing practice and establish disciplinary procedures for violations of mandates. The nurse practice acts may be accessed through the Internet (National Council of State Boards of Nursing). Many states offer a test that nurses and students can take to validate their familiarity with the law. Students who were already practicing RNs took the test as an assigned exercise and commented on its usefulness in applying the laws to their practice. Nurses reported being impressed with the extent of the "rules and regulations" applicable to their practice and, although somewhat overwhelmed, they also experience a certain sense of security that there are these guidelines to follow. Comments from students follow:

> **Nurse 1:** It was an excellent review and eye-opener. We cannot walk around in our practices guessing what the right thing to do is. We must

know exactly what the rules and regulations are and not depend on others to make sure we're following those regulations. When we're up in that courtroom, it will be us individually on that stand, defending our professional actions. Your head nurse, administrator, or colleague is not going to be able to sit on that seat with you. I definitely realize that I need to take responsibility for my practice as a nurse, and a major component of that responsibility is knowing the nurse practice act and all other related information inside out.

Nurse 2: I agree that this exercise was very beneficial. It has also raised some issues about what I know about nursing. It has helped me come to realize that nursing is not just clinical practice but it is also using the laws that govern our practice. I have now also begun to wonder who has failed us all. Is it ourselves or our governing body that we are not better versed in this information? So much of our school years are spent on assessment, planning, implementation, and evaluation of others, and little time is spent on teaching us how to safeguard and protect ourselves and our patients. I'm shocked that so little information about this is known by us.

Nurse 3: This was a reality check as to the laws and regulations that govern our practices. I will become more informed and share this information with the rest of my coworkers. I am glad we were assigned this reading. Had we not, how would we have known? I will now become more conscientious about my daily actions and the decisions I make and help others to do the same. I also took this opportunity to allow my coworkers to do the test as an educational exercise. We all felt the same way that we needed to review some more. It was definitely a worthwhile exercise. I asked one of my supervisors about these questions, and I guess she felt the same way the other coworkers felt. The questions made her realize how much she has forgotten over the years and how important it is to keep your professional practice updated.

Nurse 4: The problem is that we do not read it everyday, so we forget what it is all about. If we were to be mandated to read it every so often like any other competency, we would be more knowledgeable. Like they say "If you don't use it, you lose it," and in this case it could be very dangerous for not only our patients but for us professionally. I feel that we should have some kind of review with this at our institution. We do our competencies yearly. I feel that this should be added on! I made this suggestion to the nursing education department at my institution. Maybe even to possibly add it on to our newsletter!

Ethics

Ethics may be considered as a set of principles of right and wrong conduct that is used as a reference when making decisions about how one ought to act. Ethical behavior is closely associated with morals. The difference between the two is that morals generally refer to personal beliefs and cultural values on what is right and wrong, whereas ethics stresses the way one should act and serves as guides for professional actions.

One of the criteria of a profession is that there is a code of ethics that the members of the profession agree upon and acknowledge (Flexner, 1915). Becoming a professional nurse entails a knowledge of and commitment to follow the Code of Ethics established by the American Nurses Association (American Nurses Association, 2001). The nursing profession's first code of ethics was adopted in 1893 in the form of the Nightingale Pledge. The most recent revision of the Code of Ethics for Nurses was published by the American Nurses Association in 2001. The Code of Ethics, along with the other appendices listed below, relates to professional expectations and rights of patients. These guidelines are recommended references for each nurse and should be readily accessible (see Appendix A, The Belmont Report: Ethical Principles and Guidelines for the Protection of Human Subjects of Research, National Institutes of Health; Appendix B, Nurses Codes of Ethics With Interpretive Statements; Appendix C, The Patient Care Partnership: Understanding Expectations, Rights and Responsibilities, formerly the Patients' Bill of Rights; Appendix D, The American Nurses Association's Bill of Rights for Registered Nurses; and Appendix E, Nursing's Social Policy Statement). See Boxes 8–1, 8–2, 8–3, 8–4, and 8–5.

Ethics and Human Centered Nursing

Ethics, as with all aspects of human centered nursing, concerns the uniqueness of the individual and the principle of self-determination. As part of the human centered quality of uniqueness, people share certain aspects of human nature that

Box 8–1 | Nurses Code of Ethics With Interpretive Statements (ANA, 2001)

The Code of Ethics for nurses serves the following purposes:
It is a succinct statement of the ethical obligations and duties of every individual who enters the nursing profession.
It is the profession's nonnegotiable ethical standard.
It is an expression of nursing's own understanding of its commitment to society. (p. 5)

Box 8–2 | Basic Ethical Principles

The expression "basic ethical principles" refers to those general judgments that serve as a basic justification for the many particular ethical prescriptions and evaluations of human actions.
United States Government Department of Health and Human Services
http://www.hhs.gov/ohrp/humansubjects/guidance/belmont.htm:
2006-05-08:1006

Box 8–3 | The Patient Care Partnership: Understanding Expectations, Rights and Responsibilities

The patient care partnership proposes that health care professionals are committed to meeting the health needs of patients and families in all their ethnic, religious and economic diversity. The document explains some of the basics about how patients and their families can expect to be treated and what the professionals will need from patients and families in order to provide quality care (American Hospital Association, 2003).

Box 8–4 | Nurses Bill of Rights (ANA, 2001)

To maximize the contributions nurses make to society, it is necessary to protect the dignity and autonomy of nurses in the workplace. To that end, the American Nurses Association has delineated rights to be afforded to every nurse.

Box 8–5 | Nursing's Social Policy Statement (ANA, 2003)

[The social policy statement] expresses the social contract between society and the profession of nursing. It includes a definition of professional nursing, descriptions of professional nursing and its knowledge base, and brief descriptions of the scope of professional nursing practice and the methods by which the profession is regulated. (p. 1)

constitute their "ethical" position vis-à-vis the world. One's ethical position vis-à-vis the world is manifested in thinking, making choices, and taking responsibility for those choices. In particular, nurses participating in a human centered practice bring to each occasion a humanistically and existentially grounded way of thinking intended to make things better for everyone present. This follows from the Aristotelian idea of practical wisdom, which is a quality of a human centered nurse.

Following from this thought is the fact that most of the guides for professional conduct in nursing have to do with the way people interact with each other for some "good" intention. Ethics and morals have a contextual nature, and it is possible for people to have a professional moral or ethical set of behaviors unique to a way of thinking about life and health that are inconsistent with their personal ones. This is particularly true in nursing, where the health concerns of patients are often of a very intimate nature. The behavior of one to another is taken to be good or bad based on (1) the individual and cultural perception of the actor, (2) who is being acted upon, and (3) the context of the lived-in world in which the behavior is occurring at the particular time when it is occurring. Because individual and cultural biases can affect an individual's interpretation of what is "good" or "bad," "right" or "wrong," it is important that nurses be aware of their own beliefs and values and become familiar with the basic overlying ethical principals that are the foundation of nursing practice.

Within the interactions of nurses with patients, the practice of ethical decision making occurs thousands of times each day, as a necessary accompaniment to professional health-care delivery in institutions, communities, and homes. Hence, within nursing practice there must be an active process of reflective interpretation and practical wisdom that takes place within the experiences of every nurse (Woods, 1999). This requirement for reflection and interpretation is consistent with the human centered nursing model.

Background and Definitions in Ethics Important for Human Centered Nursing

Ethics requires understanding some basic definitions:

- Values: Beliefs strongly held about truth, beauty, worth; the way one lives one's life, derived from experience.

- Morals: Generally accepted customs of conduct and right living in a society and the individual's actions in relation to these rules of society.

- Ethics: Professional rules of conduct, rightness or wrongness of actions, goodness or badness of motives and ends of action; honest and honorable: Is this right? For whom? Is it responsible?

- Ethical principles: Respect—value of individuality and human rights; Autonomy—addresses personal freedom and self-determination; Beneficence—actions should promote and maximize the good; Nonmaleficence—does no harm (corollary of beneficence); Veracity—tell the truth; Fidelity—keeping one's promises and commitments; Justice—people should be treated fairly and equally.

These basic definitions provide material for initial discussions of ethical principles. More definitions of these principles are available at the Web sites for the National Commission for the Protection of Human Subjects of Biomedical and Behavioral Research and its institutional review board (IRB) (Belmont Report:

Ethics and Scholarship

The discussion of ethics would not be complete, especially in the academic setting, without including the application of ethically grounded principles to scholarship. This includes a commitment to hard work, developing the ability to think for oneself through the application of scholarly methods of inquiry, and the analysis and presentation of derived evidence or data that add knowledge to the body of works in the nursing literature. This way of thinking encourages students to uphold high standards in their studies, thereby affirming the value and integrity of their degrees and credentials and recognizing their services to the community. This approach to ethical scholarship is consistent with an omnipresent emphasis on ethical standards of practice in everyday nursing.

http://www.hhs.gov/ohrp/humansubjects/guidance/belmont.htm). Each academic institution has an IRB that provides extensive information on ethical principles (see Appendix A).

Case Studies: Ethics in the Classroom and Clinic

The following case study exercises provide opportunities for learning and applying ethical standards of practice as well as the mandates of the nurse practice acts. They offer situations for reflecting on and understanding ethics and ethical decision making in the context of nursing practice. Students are confronted with situations where they must struggle with competing ethical principles and personal biases. The particular case studies presented begin with a famous historical case that affords the comfort of some distance. The second case moves to a practical clinical situation that asks students to struggle with what they would do ethically and legally. The third case confronts the student with tensions that may exist between personal beliefs and values and professional ethical principles. These exercises involve not only personal reflection and deliberation but also dialogue and debate with others using references to relevant professional guidelines. Three case studies involve:

- The Tuskegee research project
- An aberrant surgeon
- A 7-year old-boy with cancer who wishes to die

Case Study One: The Tuskegee Research Project

Students watch a 45-minute video (Graubard, A., 1993) that describes the events of the Tuskegee syphilis study. In this country, in the 1940s, the Tuskegee syphilis study used disadvantaged, rural black men to study the untreated course of the disease as compared with white males. At the start of the study, penicillin had not yet been discovered as a cure for syphilis, so the researchers were not withholding an effective treatment from the black men. When penicillin later became an effective cure, researchers did deprive these black men of the treatment in order not to interrupt the research project. A key member of the research team involved in the Tuskegee project was one black nurse, Eunice Rivers, who worked with the subjects throughout the project and helped to ensure their continued participation.

Students were asked to reflect on the way Nurse Rivers conducted herself both in getting people to participate in the research project and keeping them in it after a cure for syphilis was discovered. Prior to the viewing, students are given

assignments that familiarize them with the ANA Nurses' Code of Ethics, nurse practice act of their state, and the Patient's Bill of Rights. They are instructed that as they
view or read about this study, the details are not as important as their experience or
reaction to what is being depicted.

Expected Outcomes

Students express their positions on Nurse Rivers' actions and how she did or did
not respond appropriately to the trust and affection offered by the patients.
Students give their own commentary and discuss with other classmates. It is
through these dialogues that they are challenged to consider alternative interpretations, support their own views, and articulate what they would do in a similar situation. Students derive and support arguments for the ethical framework within
which Nurse Rivers operated. The students consider and comment on how the
actions of Nurse Rivers influenced their own sense of ethical responsibility toward
patients in relation to their understanding of the Nurses' Code of Ethics and
patients' rights. Students recognize the contextual nature of ethics and relate it to
the current social and political climate, research practices, institutional organization, and professional practices.

Observed Outcomes

The following are responses from students.

> **Carol:** As I live each day, I strive to be ethical both in my life and pro-
> fessional practices. The film on the Tuskegee Project angered me for
> many reasons; all of them were ethical issues. The men involved in the
> study were lied to, mistreated, uninformed, and denied their right to
> medical care. Nurse Rivers blindly followed the instructions of her supe-
> riors while ignoring all of the very important concepts we hold today.
> The men were not informed of a cure, nor were they consulted during
> the plan of treatment. Nurse Rivers did not feel she should be held
> accountable for her actions; rather, she empowered herself with her
> incantations of the extensive measures she took to keep these men
> uninformed and participating in the study. I think we will all agree that
> the idea of pursuing the greatest good for these men was ignored. The
> only thing I can say in defense of Nurse Rivers is that some ethics are
> contextual and change over time. What was acceptable in Nurse Rivers'
> time may not be ethically acceptable in my time. And what is ethically

acceptable practice today may be frowned upon as totally barbaric practices in the future.

Fran: There was a great injustice perpetrated against poor black men in the Tuskegee Project. The men were never told that they were participating in a research project. A black nurse named Mrs. Rivers recruited the poor black men for the physicians. These men trusted her with their health-care needs, and she betrayed them. When she found out that the physicians had no intent to treat the men, she did nothing. She did not attempt to advocate for her clients. The years went by, and penicillin was discovered as a cure for the disease. The men were never treated or given the opportunity to seek treatment. Instead, they were left to degenerate under the ravages of tertiary syphilis and to transmit it to their significant others for 40 years.

Case Study Two: An Aberrant Surgeon

This exercise considers the behavior of a surgeon who does not follow hospital policies for required pre-surgery examination of his patients and tries to implicate the attending nurse in his questionable practices. Students are expected to comment on what the nurse did in response to the situation and what they might do. Students may bring in similar experiences from their practice.

In a small, rural hospital, the chief surgeon had a habit of not taking a history from and not giving a physical examination to patients before surgery. The hospital's policy was that the nurse had to sign a paper stating what preoperative preparation was done, including whether the surgeon had done the history and physical examination. She tried signing "not done" and was rebuked by the surgeon, who told her that this action was legally dangerous to him and to the hospital. The nurse decided that the best approach was to call the surgeon after each client was admitted for surgery to remind him about the history and physical. Each time he told her, "It's been dictated." Most of the time it had not been done (Guido, 1997).

Expected Outcomes

Students write reflections on the situation that addresses the ethical status of the actions of the nurse and that describe what they would do and why. Students may support their answers with paraphrased references to specific laws, rights, codes, ethical principles, etc.

Observed Outcomes

Zola: How can the doctor justify not doing a history and physical exam on a patient that he's planning to operate on? How can the nurse not act on this deviation from accepted practice? Not doing an H&P is a deviation from the standard of care that the patient is entitled to. Clearly the doctor is guilty of professional misconduct by expecting the nurse to flat-out lie by signing a piece of paper that says something was done when it was not. The idea that the doctor says that he will get in trouble unless she lies about what has and has not been done is absurd. What's wrong with this nurse? Is she afraid of the surgeon? She is not acting in the best interest of her patient, nor is she conducting herself in an ethical manner in relation to her patients or herself. The patient is at tremendous risk. Instead of trying to find ways around the situation in order to accommodate this doctor's habits, she should have chosen to do the right thing for her patients. She knew the patient could have died. The welfare of the patient was not the primary concern for the nurse, and it should have been.

Yvette: As the nurse involved, I would be negligent in my duty owed to the patient by allowing the surgery to be performed without following hospital policy. My code of ethics states that my primary commitment is to my patient and not to the attending doctor.

In keeping with the Patient's Bill of Rights, I would enquire whether the patient is aware of the risks and benefits of the procedure to be done and if there are any advance directives. I would refuse to sign off on the surgical checklist and would not send the patient to the OR until the H&P is placed in the chart. Further, I would notify the head nurse of the chief surgeon's practice. I would request that a memo be issued on the hospital's policies and procedures relating to surgeries, since I am responsible to establish conditions conducive to the provision of quality health care, and consistent with the profession. In the interest of the effective functioning of the hospital, I would request a speedy resolution to the existing crisis. Within the ethical decision-making framework, it is necessary that dilemmas be resolved immediately so as not to impact negatively on the patients.

Case Study 3: A 7-Year-Old Boy With Cancer Who Wishes to Die

The third case presents a situation in which nurses confront the tensions that can exist between personal beliefs and values and professional ethics. The case involves a 7-year-old child dying of cancer. The child expressed his desire to die rather than go through the pain of hopeless therapies that would only prolong his life for a brief period. The child asked the nurse to stand in for him and advocate on his behalf with the institution and his father, who was against the idea. The nurse elected to advocate for the boy and describes the interactions that took place (Woods, 1999) (reprinted with permission of Sage Publications).

> There was a specific child who was dying, but he still had to undergo transfusions. There comes a point where the chemotherapy has stopped working, but what happens is because the malignancy is growing out of control you have to top them up with blood transfusions and that actually keeps them going, so it extends their life. But this child, he'd had two previous transfusions and he was coming in for a third and he could have gone on like this for another three, four months, coming in every week and having a top up. He would have it, then go home and sit around and do whatever he wanted to do. But he would have been fairly limited because he would still have been required to keep coming back, and the thing that he found really traumatic was having the needle inserted for his transfusions. And he didn't want them any more; he never liked having blood transfusions and he never liked the needles that were associated with them. So he came in for his transfusion and he got me, this is a seven-year-old remember, a little seven-year-old Maori boy, and he got me aside and he said, 'I don't want this.' Really simple seven-year-old language: 'I don't want this any more.' And so I explained to him what would happen if he didn't have it, the consequences of 'I don't want this.' And that was all this sort of stuff about instead of dying in another few months' time, you will actually die in two weeks' time and he seemed to grasp all that. And I tried to con him, like it's only one needle and all the bribery and all this corruption that you do, but he was very, very adamant that it wasn't what he wanted. And he asked me to then say to his family, which was his father who was there at the time, and to the consultant and the registrar, that this was his plan of action. Because for him it was quality of life, he didn't want to live that way. So then together [he] and I got the consultants and the doctors and the

father in and we talked to them. And there were lots of tears, and the father got really angry, and I think he got really angry because the child took control, because in actual fact the child had made a decision that this was how he wanted to end his life, rather than the father saying, 'Look I really want you to live, I really want you to have the treatment, I don't want it to end.' And the child's expectation of me was that I would be his 'back up', you know his adult. He got his way! I mean it was very traumatic for me and I needed to be really strong and to stand up to not only the father, but the consultant as well, and say this is what is needed. And I think doing things like that gives you strength (Woods, 1999).

Students will reflect on the story, identifying at least one of the moral and/or ethical dilemmas. Students will comment on the identified dilemma or address dilemmas that have occurred in their own practices or life experiences, highlighting their own personal ethical or moral position.

Expected Outcomes

Students respond in various ways to the multifaceted dilemmas and explain their responses on the basis of the existential priorities of standing in for patients, making choices, and taking responsibility for those choices. Students show an awareness of and a respect for the various codes of ethics, standards of practice, and bills of rights within the framework of their nursing practice.

Observed Outcomes

Pat: We, as nurses, acknowledge and incorporate into our practices behavioral standards that reflect our own values and beliefs, as well as those of the community which we serve, sometimes resulting in ethical dilemmas. A nurse needs an understanding of the multidimensional aspects of an ethical dilemma, including intangible human factors that make each situation unique.

Faced with the situation of a 7-year-old boy receiving painful transfusions that provided only temporary palliation and degraded his quality of life, the nurse in the story chose to advocate for his request to die. She took into account his age, the uniqueness of his situated life, his worth as a person, and the need to respect his decision to refuse treatment. He made a call to her, and she responded. He trusted her to be his support system, and she felt responsible to present his feelings and decision to his father, the doctors, and the consultants. Though this was very stress-ful for her she supported him, and he eventually had his way and was allowed to die a dignified death. Although it would have caused me dis-tress (it is always difficult to see a child die) in light of his prognosis, I would have supported his decision to die with dignity.

Robin: The story of the 7-year-old boy brings to mind an actual expe-rience that I wish to offer on this subject in order to give my take on the story, as well as to suggest that these types of situations do occur and maybe not so infrequently.

Once I had a patient who was a 10-year-old girl of average matu-rity for her age who lives with her mother. Her father died of cancer 3 years earlier. The 10-year-old girl was hospitalized due to joint pain that she had been having for over the past 6 months. She was examined by her physician and found to have lupus erythematosus, a generalized dis-ease of the tissues of the body, which can affect various organs of the body. The patient was also found to have chronic kidney disease due to the lupus. Treatment with immunosuppressive drugs would improve her kidney condition and her lupus, though even with treatment, she might not live out a normal life. The mother was told first by the physician about the diagnosis, treatment, and prognosis. She told him that she did not want him or anyone else to tell her daughter about all this. She refused to allow her to be treated with the drugs. She said when her husband learned about his cancer he was very depressed. The chemotherapy left him very sick and, despite treatment, he died from his cancer. She did not want her daughter to go through the same ordeals. She wanted her daughter told that her illness was minor and that she would outgrow it. This was a point when the physician did not know what to do. Who is the doctor's patient, and to whom is he responsible? How much should a 10-year-old child be aware of her illness and participate in the decision about her treatment? I felt bad for the mother. It appeared to me that mother needed to heal from the death of the husband, something she had not had time to do, and the daughter needed someone she could openly share her feelings and worries with. I believed that the child should be given all the available information about her disease, the side effects of the drugs, and out-comes. I strongly believed that mother needed counseling to cope with her tragedy. And every patient has a right to know about her condition.

Gwen: Nurses have a moral accountability to the patients they care for and serve. This accountability extends beyond their legal responsibility in everyday nursing situations.

Ethical issues confront nurses daily. In the story, the ethical issue encountered is the quality versus quantity of life, right to die, and children's rights. The 7-year-old Maori boy doesn't want to take the treatment because he is telling the nurse that he prefers the quality of life to the quantity. He is asking for his right as an individual to die. The question is whether he, as a child, has the right to make this decision. This puts a nurse in an ethical dilemma. In this case, when the child refuses to take the treatment and prefers to die, I would talk to the child and the father and the doctor about the child's preferences. Since it is an ethical issue and the father is not agreeing with the child, I would also consider going to the bioethics committee for consultation.

Helen: This is a very sad story of a 7-year-old child who has made a decision regarding the choice to live or die. The nurse in the story acted in a professional way with compassion and respect for her client. The nurse advocated for her patient in relation to his health, safety, and rights. The nurse acted appropriately by getting together with consultants, doctors, and the father of the child. The nurse also explained to the child what would happen if he didn't have the blood transfusions. The 7-year-old child was concerned with quality of life. When cure is no longer possible, dying people primarily need good nursing care. I would respect my patient's values and desires regarding his treatment.

Kathy: The nurse, in acting on behalf of the child, showed respect and compassion for his "inherent dignity." Although [the child was] only 7 years old, the nurse believed that his feelings were valuable. It took great courage on her part, maybe even went against her beliefs, but she endeavored to intercede on his behalf. She revealed that her primary commitment was to her patient, acted as an advocate, and protected his right to choose. Autonomy for this young child was important to his quality of life as he and only he experiences it. The nurse also collaborated with other health professionals and the father to meet her young patient's needs.

Exercising autonomy is an important need of the individual, no matter what age or stage of development they are. This translates also to an important right of the patient. The nurse was prudent enough in evaluating the child's capacity to understand his needs as he saw it in regards to this important quality-of-life issue.

She informed him in easily understood language of the consequence of his actions in regards to diagnosis, treatment, and prognosis. The patient, though young, took control and made his decision. The nurse, as the adult in the relationship, bridged the connection between the child and the other adults in his life.

The nurse acted as a caregiver that practiced nursing with this child treating him with respect and recognizing him for what he is...a human being. She was also a teacher as she explained to him in language he understood about the consequences of refusing further treatment. She was a mother substitute as she stood by him lending loyal support. She mediated between the child, his father, the doctors, and the consultant so he could maintain control and choose. She advocated for him by bringing together all the parties involved that impacted his care.

The child was clever enough to engage his nurse as a back-up. He recognized that he might be considered a minor or underage. The nurse answered his call and helped him to develop this satisfying new role, and thus his needs were met.

In this case I believe that I would have done the same as the nurse, but it would have been a difficult experience for me. I would respect his wishes and advocate fully for him, but seeing an end to such a young life would be traumatic to me and bracketing my feelings would be absolutely necessary. I would empathize with the child and his father, fight hard with the doctors and the consultant, and request spiritual guidance for those involved as needed. I would gain the courage and fight to fulfill his wish. I am also a strong advocate in obtaining optimum quality of life in end-of-life care. This would present a conflict, but I know I could never face that child if I stood by and watched while another needle was inserted in his arm. It would go against my personal and ethical values. His trust in me as his nurse would be shattered, and it would be as if I lost some essence of my personal and professional self.

Summary

Despite the fact that there are extensive guidelines for consensual and appropriate interventions in the delivery of nursing care contained in the Nurses' Code of Ethics, nurse practice acts, Nurses' Social Policy Statement, Patients' Bill of Rights, and other proprietary institutional standards, there are many occasions where nurses face value and ethical conflicts. This is primarily because of the uniqueness of each nursing occasion. Nurses are routinely called to engage in a process of ethical decision making, which entails experiential wisdom from previous nursing occasions as well as the influence of inhered values and beliefs. Nurses' set of life-world meanings will influence their chosen actions, but necessarily those actions must also be consistent with respect to their professional ethics and legal obligations. In order for nurses to fulfill these responsibilities, they must be knowledgeable about those ethics and how they relate to patients' rights.

REFERENCES

American Hospital Association. (2003). *The patient care partnership: Understanding expectations, rights and responsibilities.*

American Nurses Association. (2001). *Nurses code of ethics with interpretive statements.* Nursesbooks.org, Silver Spring, Md.

American Nurses Association. (2003). *Nursing's social policy statement.* Nursesbooks.org, Silver Spring, Md.

Flexner, A. (1915). Is social work a profession? In *Proceedings of the national conference on social work,* pp. 578–581. New York.

Graubard, A. (1993). Film: *Critical thinking in nursing: Lessons from Tuskegee.* National League of Nursing.

Guido, G.W. (1997). *Legal issues in nursing,* 2nd ed. Stamford, Conn.: Appleton & Lange.

United States Government Department of Health and Human Services. *Belmont report.* Available at http://www.hhs.gov/ohrp/humansubjects/guidance/belmont.htm

Woods, M. (1999). A nursing ethic: The moral voice of experienced nurses. *Nursing Ethics,* 6(5), 423. Sage Publications.

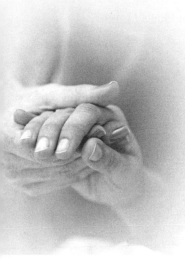

Chapter 9

Learning and Teaching From a Human Centered Practice Perspective

I t does not matter whether we are students, teachers, or working nurses; we are all engaged in a continuous process of learning. There are many learning strategies available. Some of these strategies address the learner, some address the teacher, and some address both student and teacher. Some are highly theoretical elaborations on the processes of learning and teaching, and others give detailed procedural guidelines.

Many of the offerings in the literature on learning suggest alternative or augmentative pedagogical strategies to the classical classroom-lecture, note-taking, rote-memorization, test-taking format. Many propose some form of participatory model of teaching and learning, and others argue that the implementation of technology can lead to improved learning outcomes.

In particular, Flowers (2001) makes a lucid argument for the use of high-tech media in the learning process, especially in scientific and engineering subject areas, such as electromagnetism and calculus. Flowers' reasoning may have application in nursing and health care in such subject areas as pharmacology, microbiology, and anatomy and physiology as well as in reviews for licensure examinations, which for the most part are objective and concrete.

On the other hand, Lave (1996) argues that it is crucial to frame the study of education within explicit accounts of its different theoretical perspectives. He emphasizes that learning is the identity-making life project of individuals and evolves from participation in socially situated engagements in communities of practice. The style of learning suggested in this chapter enables the bringing forth into awareness or presence those very identity-making phenomena that, by definition, evolve from participation in socially situated engagements in communities of practice and reflective contemplation; in other words, thinking.

These pedagogical strategies suggest that the goal or desire of all learning and teaching activities is to bring into awareness and gain fluency with some thing, idea, or image that was not present before the learning took place. This final chapter offers a way of learning and teaching that will help the reader gain a deeper understanding of and fluency with the ideas introduced in this book. The pedagogical approach is succinctly conceptualized to show the way—"to move" or "to be moved" toward learning. The style of learning and teaching suggested here is particularly suited to human centered nursing because it aids in discovering what it is that lies within and outside our selves—a fundamental requirement of living in the world with others as people are moved to become as much as they can be and to help others do the same.

Thinking and Learning

Martin Heidegger believed that the process of learning is related to, and resides in, a larger framework of a certain type of thinking. In his essay "What Is Called Thinking?" excerpted from his lecture series (Heidegger, 1993), he describes how he guided his students to what is meant by thinking from a perspective other than the type of thinking that encompasses calculating, figuring, planning, or problem solving. These forms of mental processes are usually associated with the scientific and the demonstrable. They are found in acquiring or implementing useful scientific and technical knowledge, practiced in such areas as business, mathematics, engineering, and technology.

We have adopted the teachings of Heidegger, who spent most of his career as a teacher. Cited are two references, Heidegger (1993) and Richardson (2003), which were selected as relevant for teaching and learning and for their insight into Heidegger's philosophy of learning. This chapter in no way qualifies as an exposition of Heidegger's work. It is, rather, an attempt to inquire into some of Heidegger's thoughts on teaching, learning, and thinking and to offer them as possibilities for formulating a philosophy of learning appropriate to nursing.

In health care, and in nursing in particular, this type of thinking is needed for the acquisition and implementation of technical knowledge and practical skills. Indeed, many nursing skills require technological, mathematical, engineering, and business competencies. Furthermore, many nursing topics and skills, such as pharmacology, physical assessment, microbiology, taking blood pressure, giving injections, and calculating medication dosage, depend on a calculative and deductive form of thinking. These topics and skills are unquestionably essential for licensure, certification, and certainly for safety.

There is more to nursing, however, than calculating and manipulating scientific and technical knowledge. A mode of thinking as a prelude to learning is needed that is appropriate to the nursing occasion represented by one person calling out to another for recognition and help. For this reason, a conception of thinking is offered that follows Heidegger's teachings on the subject.

What is Thinking and its Relevance for Nursing?

Heidegger (1993) indicates that the very nature of "being" is consistent with "thinking." These two attributes of human existence are complementary and are embedded within the existential imperative that human beings have the unique ability and responsibility to think and make choices and to take responsibility for those choices.

Heidegger (1993) declared that "thinking holds to the coming of what has been, and is remembrance. It is a question raised on all sides and always with a sense of urgency, it hinges on nothing less than the survival of the species man and the planet earth" (p. 307). What Heidegger means by the "coming of what has been" and "remembrance," or recollection, in a very broad sense is a process of "presencing," bringing into, or letting come into, presence, or awareness, some thing, impression, phenomenon, or experience. This entails making it available for questioning, wondering, awe, revealing, interpretation, from which some essence or truth may be derived. From these existential truths spring forth the values that give meaning to and enhance the lived-in-world, nursing practices, and scholarship, including moral and ethical standpoints.

What comes to presence often comes through the senses, and it offers access to a better remembering and understanding of its essential nature than that which is derived through a process of rational thought (Heidegger, 1993; Proust, 1922). Proust (1922) gives an example of how past events can be brought into present consciousness through the senses. In his most admired work, *Remembrance of Things*

Past (1922), he explained that past experiences can be brought into current consciousness by reflecting on symbols such as the madeleine cakes. In a scene from *Swann's Way*, the first volume, a madeleine cake (a small, rich cookie-like pastry) enables Marcel to experience the past completely as a simultaneous part of his present existence. He summed up the experience by writing:

> And suddenly the memory returns. The taste was that of the little crumb of madeleine which on Sunday mornings at Combray (because on those mornings I did not go out before church-time), when I went to say good day to her in her bedroom, my aunt Leonie used to give me, dipping it first in her own cup of real or of lime-flower tea. The sight of the little madeleine had recalled nothing to my mind before I tasted it; perhaps because I had so often seen such things in the interval, without tasting them, on the trays in pastry-cooks' windows, that their image had dissociated itself from those Combray days to take its place among others more recent; perhaps because of those memories, so long abandoned and put out of mind, nothing now survived, everything was scattered; the forms of things, including that of the little scallop-shell of pastry, so richly sensual under its severe, religious folds, were either obliterated or had been so long dormant as to have lost the power of expansion which would have allowed them to resume their place in my consciousness. But when from a long-distant past nothing subsists, after the people are dead, after the things are broken and scattered, still, alone, more fragile, but with more vitality, more unsubstantial, more persistent, more faithful, the smell and taste of things remain poised a long time, like souls, ready to remind us, waiting and hoping for their moment, amid the ruins of all the rest; and bear unfaltering, in the tiny and almost impalpable drop of their essence, the vast structure of recollection.
>
> And once I had recognized the taste of the crumb of madeleine soaked in her decoction of lime-flowers which my aunt used to give me (although I did not yet know and must long postpone the discovery of why this memory made me so happy) immediately the old grey house upon the street, where her room was, rose up like the scenery of a theatre to attach itself to the little pavilion, opening on to the garden, which had been built out behind it for my parents (the isolated panel which until that moment had been all that I could see); and

with the house the town, from morning to night and in all weathers, the Square where I was sent before luncheon, the streets along which I used to run errands, the country roads we took when it was fine. And just as the Japanese amuse themselves by filling a porcelain bowl with water and steeping in it little crumbs of paper which until then are without character or form, but, the moment they become wet, stretch themselves and bend, take on colour and distinctive shape, become flowers or houses or people, permanent and recognisable, so in that moment all the flowers in our garden and in M. Swann's park, and the water-lilies on the Vivonne and the good folk of the village and their little dwellings and the parish church and the whole of Combray and of its surroundings, taking their proper shapes and growing solid, sprang into being, town and gardens alike, from my cup of tea.

Sense Perception as Aesthesis

Coming through the senses refers to that type of sense perception that the Greeks called *aesthesis.* Aesthesis is the idea of sensual apperception giving access to, and awareness of, some universal or primordial truths of existence. This is congruent with the movement from presence to thinking to essence or truth (or presence to thinking to learning) in the model of learning being presented here.

As an example, consider the sense of touch in all of its nuances as it relates to nursing. According to Aristotle in his *De Anima,* touch is the primary form of sense (Aristotle, trans. 1931). Buber (1965), in his discussion of the I/thou phenomenon in intersubjective relationships, speaks of the primacy of touch as coincidence and correspondence with our knowledge of universal truths (see the kitchen conference in Chapter 3 in the dialogues with Paterson and Zderad).

Technology Versus Thinking

Because the spirit of the time *(Zeitgeist)* is profoundly influenced by technology, people must recognize the potential threat that technological advances pose to thinking in general and particularly the type of thinking discussed in this book. People must be aware of the extent to which the tools of technology conceal possibilities of informing human styles of thinking, deliberating, and making choices in general as well as how nurses in particular present themselves to and interact with patients, families, and other health-care professionals.

The reflections of nursing students in an RN-to-BSN program exemplify this threat:

> As a practicing registered nurse, I appreciate the new technologies that assist me with my nightly duties, but on more than one occasion I have come to realize that some of the instruments remove the therapeutic touch from my care activities. When I have assessed patients' blood pressure using the manual instead of the automatic blood pressure cuff, palpating the radial or brachial pulse, patients have held onto my hand making various comments, such as "your hands are so nice and warm," or they would rub my hand. This never happened when I used the automatic blood pressure machines as it was a wrap, or the press of a button, and blood pressure and pulse reading would be on the screen. Sometimes as nurses, because of the various duties we have to perform during our shift, we do not take time to touch or speak to our patients. I have realized that most of my patients, especially the elderly, value this touch. Because of this I now assess my patients' blood pressure when possible with the manual cuff and palpate their radial or brachial pulse.

Another nursing student writes:

> I think that my nursing care function is being stretched to a level where you cannot see the patient, only the computer screen and all the red and green lights around him. The sound that beckons is not the scared voice of Mr. John Doe but the alarm on the machine that quickens my step while I remind myself to check the want ads for ads seeking 'nurses to do nursing.'

This motif of technology is called *technicity*. Technicity is the manner in which entities-in-the-world, including human beings, are experienced as objects that are available and subject to control and exploitation (Heidegger, 1993; Richardson, 2003; Sheehan, 1999). In today's world of accelerated technologization, there is a pervasive tension between thinking and technology.

Henry David Thoreau was one of the first to notice the dangers of the phenomenon of technicity. He expressed his disdain for the way his neighbors seemed to be infatuated with the possession of "things," whether or not these things contributed to an experience of a good life. He lamented the lack of initiative and innovation on the part of people who were willing merely to acquire and accumulate things instead of engaging in the self-satisfying project of doing or creating for themselves.

The practice of just taking what is available, whether it has any real utility or consequence for a good life, was accelerated by the introduction of new technology that began to proliferate during the Industrial Revolution. The exorbitant proliferation of technology signaled a change in the concept of technology from one of defining man's relationship to his tools as "man-using-tool" to one of "tool-using-man." Accordingly, "...men have become the tool of their tools (Thoreau, 1985, p. 352)."

It was this blind acquiescence to the technological imperative without concern for its consequences that Thoreau feared and to which he objected. He argued that "no doubt another may also think for me; but it is not therefore desirable that he should do so to the exclusion of my thinking for myself" (p. 359).

A hundred years later, Heidegger reiterated the warnings of Thoreau, saying that "everywhere we remain unfree and chained to technology....But we are delivered over to it in the worst possible way when we regard it as something neutral" (1993, pp. 311–312). He insisted that thinking was the way out of this dilemma, specifically the thinking as defined in this chapter and adopted in the human centered nursing model.

Others followed Heidegger's lead. For example, Wills (2004) warned that if people do not change their way of thinking about technology, "...we will be unable to recognize technology or begin to account for its increasing direction of our movements and lives...nor will we be able to set about resisting or responding to it" (p. 51). Beardsworth (1998) worried about "the evermore explicit [technologization] of the world, and how this process explicitly defies the syntheses of human imagination and invention" (p. 70). He asserts that people must engage in a process of thinking and developing an understanding of technicity in order to clarify the political and ethical issues that arise from it. Kleiman and Kleiman (2007) elaborated on the relationship among technology, technicity, and thinking in a Heideggerian sense. The Kleiman position is not to argue that technology is good or bad but rather to point out that technology as technicity may set aside or push into the background of dialogue about nursing some of the precepts of human centered nursing, such as being-with, becoming as much as one can be, making choices, and taking responsibility for those choices.

Creating Out of What Has Come Into Presence

Thinking in the manner described in this chapter always entails inquiry and wonder, which inspire acts of creation from what has been brought into current consciousness or awareness. This is termed creative learning. Children at work in a kindergarten class illustrate this idea. With very basic elements—for example, blocks and finger paints—children's imaginations are stimulated, and their hidden potentials are uncovered and revealed through their creations. It is through this creative process that they begin to learn, such as the properties of structures in stacking, balance, and center of gravity. In the case of paints, they learn how colors can be mixed and contrasted to create certain moods.

It may be difficult to recognize what the resultant creation is because sometimes what is created with blocks, finger paints, tinker toys, and imagination demands interrogation—the question 'what is it?' It is through this process of inquiry and wonder that the creator struggles to articulate and give a name to the creation. This questioning may lead to the creation taking on some form of identity, unconcealing the meanings or concepts that it symbolizes, and letting it be shared with and understood by others.

The dynamic is similar to starting with an abstract construct (experience or phenomenon) and, through reflective thought, bringing forth both the latent and obvious potentialities that offer possibilities for finding the essential nature or meaning for oneself. The nurse, as creator, presents a creation through some linguistic form or presence and offers it to and for another. Engagement in the process also provides occasions for discovering and affirming truths and values that contribute to one's identity.

Paterson and Zderad (1988) referred to this type of thinking that engenders a bringing into awareness as the way that a nurse gains access to others as a "noetic locus" or "knowing place." They stated: "I consider my greatest gifts as a human being nurse my ability to relate to other man, to wonder, search and imagine about my experience, and to create out of what I come to know. My ever developing internalized community of world thinkers dynamically interrelated with my conscious awareness of my experienced nursing realm allows my appreciation of my human gifts and the ever enrichment of myself as a 'knowing place'" (p. 37).

Teaching

The Heideggerian lessons on learning and thinking can also be applied to teaching. Hultgren (1995), who follows Heidegger's lesson, operates within a theoretical framework of existentialism and ontology and argues that teaching is to "let-learn" and that the teacher engages in the process as a learner. Hultgren states, "To let learn means: To prepare a space for listening that intertwines identities (self/other and self/society) in retrieval of being, a leading in itself that withdraws from teacher to being-in-teaching-together" (1995, p. 377). In this space, both student and teacher are provided the opportunity to grow and become more; in other words, the opportunity to "let learn".

Gibbs and Angelides (2004) use Heidegger's concept of "let learn" to present some important ideas related to phronesis, or practical wisdom, and being-in-the-world. Refer to Chapter 4 for a full discussion of practical wisdom and phronesis.

Gibbs and Angelides argue that experiential learning leading to phronesis, or practical wisdom, is preferable to models of learning currently in use. Jamieson (2005) relates the learning techniques used by the painter Goya, who, as a boy, was educated by the Escolapian Fathers in a monastic school. Goya was taught to rely on his own faculties, to observe, to make deductions from his personal experience, to discover the flexibility of his own mind, and to assume responsibility for assimilating as much knowledge as possible. Note the similarity to thinking, making choices, and taking responsibility for those choices.

The "letting-learn" teaching occasion entails the participation of one person with another with the goal of moving each other to an awareness or a deeper understanding of some phenomenon or uncovered potentiality. To let learn is, at the highest level of abstraction, to show students how to learn by thinking and to instill in them the value that the learning process entails.

Teachers have a responsibility to introduce to students that which is thought-provoking, that which has relevance for essential being in the world with others. Teachers need to encourage students to welcome that which challenges the usual and standard and to approach the world with an inquisitive mind that is open to the truth of what is being presented. After all, learning in nursing does not end in the classroom but is a continuous process of enhancement that carries forward in each nurse's career.

For students and practicing nurses, thinking and learning are fundamental to nursing and quality care, despite the ever-changing technological and business models that pervade every aspect of health-care institutions. According to Heidegger (1993), the urgency to continue to exercise thinking is not an option. Complacency, deference to someone or something, or rejection or subordination in any way, holds dire consequences for the human race and in particular what is known as nursing. Thus, by letting learn, the teacher sets the student on the road to learning by thinking, encouraging students to think by giving them things to think about. By learning through thinking, the student is able to uncover the truths of existence or the essential nature of being-in-the-world.

Letting Learn in the Classroom or Clinic: Authentic Presence

A key point that Heidegger made in his lectures was that in the learning process, students and teacher are of equal status. The teacher is not an elite personality who dictates what "is" to the subordinate student, who nods in acquiescence to the teacher's brilliance. Rather, because the teacher has as much to learn as the student, the teacher is a participant in the learning process and helps the student to learn "learning." Heidegger (1993) used the example of the cabinetmaker's apprentice, a person who is learning to build cabinets and similar objects under the tutelage of the master. The apprentice's project is not merely to learn how to select and use the tools necessary to cut, carve, shape, and color wood, but rather to learn how to bring forward the hidden potential of the wood in all its possibilities for transformation into furniture. The apprentice's proper learning is in bringing forth the essence (the beauty) of wood as the essence of cabinet making.

In this simple but profound example, Heidegger shows how the apprentice asserts his proper learning by bringing out the beauty of his object in its essential form. The proper place of the teacher is to guide the student in the process of learning by way of thinking in order to help the student learn learning, that is, how to bring forward the essential nature of the object of investigation or construction.

This metaphor can be carried to the nursing experience. The nurse's main concern is not learning how to select and use the stethoscope, thermometer, or blood pressure device or how to give an injection or calculate a medication dosage, although these are necessary tools and skills. Rather, the nurse is primarily concerned with bringing forth the essence of nursing. The nursing student asserts proper learning by bringing out her object as it is manifested in patient care in health, sickness, or dying. That, in its essential form, is nursing. The essential form of nursing is "being and becoming," participating with patients, families, students, and colleagues, in a process of becoming as much as one can be regardless of the situation in which one is occupied.

Before the learning process in which the teacher is a true participant can begin, the teacher must provide the space in which thinking and learning can occur. That is, the teacher must open the way into a field of potential within which students discover possibilities for thought. The teacher opens the way to thinking by assuming an attitude similar to that which she presents to patients in a clinical setting: an attitude of open and attentive apperception, without prejudice and with an awareness of the students' presence and uniqueness. The teacher is ready to listen and to hear and is willing to make a connection with each student that entails mutual respect for personal dignity, history, and current life situation.

This attitude or state-of-being is authentic presence. Moving toward authentic presence assumes that individuals have as part of their historical, cultural, and environmental identity certain values and life experiences that affect how they make decisions and how they will act and react to events and situations in which they become engaged. Some of these values will manifest readily in interactions with others. Some will lie hidden, latent or quiescent, in the depths of memory. These values need to be brought into current awareness, made present for thinking, as they hold possibilities for enabling the individual's self-actualizing potential.

Reflecting, Sharing, Learning

One of the ways to stimulate interest and participation in this process is to invite students to engage in exercises of reflection on class activities, clinic events, and readings from the literature. Sharing one's experiences is part of this process. As students uncover those values that are evoked by their awareness of, and engagement in, life's experiences, the teacher gains insight and refines and augments her own values and ethical bases.

The phenomenon of sharing intermediates the learning and presencing process, allowing what has come into presence to be brought into discourse. Not sharing what has been uncovered is the most serious of defects because sharing is a fundamental property of being and becoming in the nursing experience (Paterson & Zderad, 1976).

From a practical point of view, sharing among students can be fruitful. It brings experiences into discourse that help to illuminate their meanings and values for introspection by other nurses, and it instills a sense of community.

The following example is based on the experience of a student in a class that recently finished a group project with other students:

These people are to be commended. I was so proud to be in their company. This sharing also allowed us as students to find resources amongst ourselves. I have honestly never had an opportunity in all my years at this college to actually get to know those that struggle with me in this program. I'm thankful that I got to hear a bit about their lives and their experience as well as their gifts and downfalls. None of us is perfect, and it hasn't been easy for anyone to get to where we are. I felt a real sense of comraderie and support from my classmates. We ended on such a delightful note that I felt it really empowered me. We even came up with a slogan, "Together Everyone Accomplishes More." I will do my best to make myself available to my peers.

This reflection led to a discussion on how this commitment to struggle together can be the basis of a community of nurses helping each other to become all that each can be and all that nursing can be in this complex world of health care. When reflections such as this are shared in class, the lecture or clinic is transformed. The gathering of a group of people attending to a particular subject becomes intersubjective, an occasion of learning together where students and teacher affirm their own identity and that of others.

It is here that the idea of let-learn comes to full bloom. Here, the novice can find, develop, and shape her ideas, values, personal ethics, and conceptions of relationships with others of diverse and similar backgrounds. Here, the more experienced individuals have the opportunity to explore possibilities, to rethink their values, personal ethics, and relationships with others. For all students, there is the opportunity to locate or relocate their place in the nursing community.

Wondering about thinking and learning in a Heideggerian sense offers possibilities for both theoretical and practical conceptualization and participation in the way to learn and experience nursing. Nurses take part in learning, valuing their scholarship and nursing experiences, becoming more as persons, helping others to grow, and finally, enjoying a nursing career marked by self-actualization and personal and professional growth and satisfaction.

REFERENCES

Aristotle. (350 BC/1931). *De anima*, trans. J. A. Smith. Accessed November 13, 2006, from http://etext.library.adelaide.edu.au/mirror/classics.mit.edu/Aristotle/soul.mb.txt

Beardsworth, R. (1998). *Thinking technicity: Cultural values.* Blackwell Publishers Ltd.

Buber, M. (1965). *The knowledge of man.* New York: Harper & Row.

Flowers, W. (2001). *New media's impact on education strategies.* Accessed April 15, 2007, from http://www.educause.edu/LibraryDetailPage/666?ID=FFPIU016

Gibbs, P., & Angelides, P. (2004). Accreditation of knowledge as being-in-the-world. *Journal of Education and Work,* 17(3), 333–346.

Heidegger, M. (1993). *Basic writings* , 2nd ed. Edited by D. F. Krell. San Francisco: Harper Collins.

Hultgren, F. (1995). The phenomenology of "doing" phenomenology: The experience of teaching and learning together. *Human Studies,* 18(4), 371–388.

Jamieson, A. (2005). An essay on the life and work of Francisco Goya. *Work-Based Learning in Primary Care,* 3(3), 236–252.

Kleiman, S., & Kleiman, A. (2007). Technicity in nursing and the dispensation of thinking. *Nursing Economic$*, 25(3).

Lave, J. (1996). Teaching, as learning, in practice. *Mind, Culture, and Activity: An International Journal*, 3(3), 149–164.

Paterson, J., & Zderad, L. (1976). *Humanistic nursing.* New York: John Wiley & Sons.

Paterson, J., & Zderad, L. (1988). *Humanistic nursing.* New York: National League for Nursing.

Proust. M. (1922). *Swann's Way*, Volume 1 of *Remembrance of Things Past*, Trans. Scott-Moncrieff, C. K. New York: Henry Holt and Company. Accessed November 16, 2007, from http://www.gutenberg.org/wtext/7178

Richardson, W. (2003). *Through phenomenology to thought.* New York: Fordham University Press.

Sheehan, T. (1999). *Martin Heidegger, A companion to the philosophers*, ed. Robert L. Arrington. Oxford and Oxford, UK: Blackwell, pp. 288–297.

Thoreau, H. (1985). Prose works: *A week on the Concord and Merrimack rivers; Walden, or, life in the woods; The Maine woods.* Cape Cod, N.Y.: Literary Classics of the United States.

Wills, D. (2004). Thinking back: Towards technology via dorsality. *Parallax* 10(3), 36–52.

Permissions

Excerpts from:

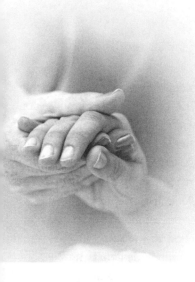

Appendix A

The Belmont Report: Ethical Principles and Guidelines for the Protection of Human Subjects of Research, National Institutes of Health

The National Commission for the Protection of Human Subjects of Biomedical and Behavioral Research

April 18, 1979

AGENCY: Department of Health, Education, and Welfare.

ACTION: Notice of Report for Public Comment.

SUMMARY: On July 12, 1974, the National Research Act (Pub. L. 93-348) was signed into law, thereby creating the National Commission for the Protection of Human Subjects of Biomedical and Behavioral Research. One of the charges to the Commission was to identify the basic ethical principles that should underlie the conduct of biomedical and behavioral research involving human subjects and to develop guidelines which should be followed to assure that such research is conducted in accordance with those principles. In carrying out the above, the Commission was directed to consider: (i) the boundaries between biomedical and behavioral research and the accepted and routine practice of medicine, (ii) the role of assessment of risk-benefit criteria in the determination of the appropriateness of research involving human subjects, (iii) appropriate guidelines for the selection of human subjects for participation in such research and (iv) the nature and definition of informed consent in various research settings.

The Belmont Report attempts to summarize the basic ethical principles identified by the Commission in the course of its deliberations. It is the outgrowth of an intensive four-day period of discussions that were held in February 1976 at the

Smithsonian Institution's Belmont Conference Center supplemented by the monthly deliberations of the Commission that were held over a period of nearly four years. It is a statement of basic ethical principles and guidelines that should assist in resolving the ethical problems that surround the conduct of research with human subjects. By publishing the Report in the Federal Register, and providing reprints upon request, the Secretary intends that it may be made readily available to scientists, members of Institutional Review Boards, and Federal employees. [...]

Unlike most other reports of the Commission, the Belmont Report does not make specific recommendations for administrative action by the Secretary of Health, Education, and Welfare. Rather, the Commission recommended that the Belmont Report be adopted in its entirety, as a statement of the Department's policy. The Department requests public comment on this recommendation. [...]

Ethical Principles and Guidelines for Research Involving Human Subjects

Scientific research has produced substantial social benefits. It has also posed some troubling ethical questions. Public attention was drawn to these questions by reported abuses of human subjects in biomedical experiments, especially during the Second World War. During the Nuremberg War Crime Trials, the Nuremberg code was drafted as a set of standards for judging physicians and scientists who had conducted biomedical experiments on concentration camp prisoners. This code became the prototype of many later codes* intended to assure that research involving human subjects would be carried out in an ethical manner.

The codes consist of rules, some general, others specific, that guide the investigators or the reviewers of research in their work. Such rules often are inadequate to cover complex situations; at times they come into conflict, and they are frequently difficult to interpret or apply. Broader ethical principles will provide a basis on which specific rules may be formulated, criticized and interpreted.

---

*Since 1945, various codes for the proper and responsible conduct of human experimentation in medical research have been adopted by different organizations. The best known of these codes are the Nuremberg Code of 1947, the Helsinki Declaration of 1964 (revised in 1975), and the 1971 Guidelines (codified into Federal Regulations in 1974) issued by the U.S. Department of Health, Education, and Welfare. Codes for the conduct of social and behavioral research have also been adopted, the best known being that of the American Psychological Association, published in 1973. Retrieved from: http://ohsr.od.nih.gov/guidelines/belmont.html on October 16, 2007

Three principles, or general prescriptive judgments, that are relevant to research involving human subjects are identified in this statement. Other principles may also be relevant. These three are comprehensive, however, and are stated at a level of generalization that should assist scientists, subjects, reviewers and interested citizens to understand the ethical issues inherent in research involving human subjects. These principles cannot always be applied so as to resolve beyond dispute particular ethical problems. The objective is to provide an analytical framework that will guide the resolution of ethical problems arising from research involving human subjects.

This statement consists of a distinction between research and practice, a discussion of the three basic ethical principles, and remarks about the application of these principles.

Part A: Boundaries Between Practice & Research

A Boundaries Between Practice and Research
It is important to distinguish between biomedical and behavioral research, on the one hand, and the practice of accepted therapy on the other, in order to know what activities ought to undergo review for the protection of human subjects of research. The distinction between research and practice is blurred partly because both often occur together (as in research designed to evaluate a therapy) and partly because notable departures from standard practice are often called "experimental" when the terms "experimental" and "research" are not carefully defined.

For the most part, the term "practice" refers to interventions that are designed solely to enhance the well-being of an individual patient or client and that have a reasonable expectation of success. The purpose of medical or behavioral practice is to provide diagnosis, preventive treatment or therapy to particular individuals....By contrast, the term "research" designates an activity designed to test an hypothesis, permit conclusions to be drawn, and thereby to develop or contribute to generalizable knowledge (expressed, for example, in theories, principles, and statements of relationships). Research is usually described in a formal protocol that sets forth an objective and a set of procedures designed to reach that objective.

When a clinician departs in a significant way from standard or accepted practice, the innovation does not, in and of itself, constitute research. The fact that a procedure is "experimental," in the sense of new, untested or different, does not automatically place it in the category of research. Radically new procedures of this description should, however, be made the object of formal research at an early stage in order to determine whether they are safe and effective. Thus, it is the responsibility of medical practice committees, for example, to insist that a major innovation be incorporated into a formal research project....

Research and practice may be carried on together when research is designed to evaluate the safety and efficacy of a therapy. This need not cause any confusion regarding whether or not the activity requires review; the general rule is that if there is any element of research in an activity, that activity should undergo review for the protection of human subjects.

Part B: Basic Ethical Principles

B. Basic Ethical Principles

The expression "basic ethical principles" refers to those general judgments that serve as a basic justification for the many particular ethical prescriptions and evaluations of human actions. Three basic principles, among those generally accepted in our cultural tradition, are particularly relevant to the ethics of research involving human subjects: the principles of respect of persons, beneficence and justice.

1. **Respect for Persons**—Respect for persons incorporates at least two ethical convictions: first, that individuals should be treated as autonomous agents, and second, that persons with diminished autonomy are entitled to protection. The principle of respect for persons thus divides into two separate moral requirements: the requirement to acknowledge autonomy and the requirement to protect those with diminished autonomy.

   An autonomous person is an individual capable of deliberation about personal goals and of acting under the direction of such deliberation. To respect autonomy is to give weight to autonomous persons' considered opinions and choices while refraining from obstructing their actions unless they are clearly detrimental to others. To show lack of respect for an autonomous agent is to repudiate that person's considered judgments, to deny an individual the freedom to act on those considered judgments, or to withhold information necessary to make a considered judgment, when there are no compelling reasons to do so.

   However, not every human being is capable of self-determination. The capacity for self-determination matures during an individual's life, and some individuals lose this capacity wholly or in part because of illness, mental disability, or circumstances that severely restrict liberty.

Respect for the immature and the incapacitated may require protecting them as they mature or while they are incapacitated.

Some persons are in need of extensive protection, even to the point of excluding them from activities which may harm them; other persons require little protection beyond making sure they undertake activities freely and with awareness of possible adverse consequence. The extent of protection afforded should depend upon the risk of harm and the likelihood of benefit. The judgment that any individual lacks autonomy should be periodically reevaluated and will vary in different situations.

In most cases of research involving human subjects, respect for persons demands that subjects enter into the research voluntarily and with adequate information. In some situations, however, application of the principle is not obvious. The involvement of prisoners as subjects of research provides an instructive example. On the one hand, it would seem that the principle of respect for persons requires that prisoners not be deprived of the opportunity to volunteer for research. On the other hand, under prison conditions they may be subtly coerced or unduly influenced to engage in research activities for which they would not otherwise volunteer. Respect for persons would then dictate that prisoners be protected. Whether to allow prisoners to "volunteer" or to "protect" them presents a dilemma. Respecting persons, in most hard cases, is often a matter of balancing competing claims urged by the principle of respect itself.

2. **Beneficence**—Persons are treated in an ethical manner not only by respecting their decisions and protecting them from harm, but also by making efforts to secure their well-being. Such treatment falls under the principle of beneficence. The term "beneficence" is often understood to cover acts of kindness or charity that go beyond strict obligation. In this document, beneficence is understood in a stronger sense, as an obligation. Two general rules have been formulated as complementary expressions of beneficent actions in this sense: (1) do not harm and (2) maximize possible benefits and minimize possible harms.

The Hippocratic maxim "do no harm" has long been a fundamental principle of medical ethics. Claude Bernard extended it to the realm of research, saying that one should not injure one person regardless of the benefits that might come to others. However, even avoiding harm requires learning what is harmful; and, in the process of obtaining this information, persons may be exposed to risk of harm. Further, the Hippocratic Oath requires physicians to benefit their patients "according to their best judgment." Learning what will in fact benefit may require exposing persons to risk. The problem posed by these imperatives is to decide when it is justifiable to seek certain benefits despite the risks involved, and when the benefits should be foregone because of the risks.

The obligations of beneficence affect both individual investigators and society at large, because they extend both to particular research projects and to the entire enterprise of research. In the case of particular projects, investigators and members of their institutions are obliged to give forethought to the maximization of benefits and the reduction of risk that might occur from the research investigation. In the case of scientific research in general, members of the larger society are obliged to recognize the longer-term benefits and risks that may result from the improvement of knowledge and from the development of novel medical, psychotherapeutic, and social procedures.

The principle of beneficence often occupies a well-defined justifying role in many areas of research involving human subjects. An example is found in research involving children. Effective ways of treating childhood diseases and fostering healthy development are benefits that serve to justify research involving children—even when individual research subjects are not direct beneficiaries. Research also makes it possible to avoid the harm that may result from the application of previously accepted routine practices that on closer investigation turn out to be dangerous. But the role of the principle of beneficence is not always so unambiguous. A difficult ethical problem remains, for example, about research that presents more than minimal risk without immediate prospect of direct benefit to the children involved. Some have argued that such research is inadmissible, while others have pointed out that this limit would rule out much research promising great benefit to children in the future. Here again, as with all hard cases, the different claims covered by the principle of beneficence may come into conflict and force difficult choices.

3. **Justice**—Who ought to receive the benefits of research and bear its burdens? This is a question of justice, in the sense of "fairness in distribution" or "what is deserved." An injustice occurs when some benefit to which a person is entitled is denied without good reason or when some burden is imposed unduly. Another way of conceiving the principle of justice is that equals ought to be treated equally. However, this statement requires explication. Who is equal and who is unequal? What considerations justify departure from equal distribution? Almost all commentators allow that distinctions based on experience, age, deprivation, competence, merit and position do sometimes constitute criteria justifying differential treatment for certain purposes. It is necessary, then, to explain in what respects people should be treated equally. There are several widely accepted formulations of just ways to distribute burdens and benefits. Each formulation mentions some relevant property on the basis of which burdens and benefits should be distributed. These formulations are (1) to each person an equal share, (2) to each person according to individual need, (3) to each person according to individual effort, (4) to each person according to societal contribution, and (5) to each person according to merit.

Questions of justice have long been associated with social practices such as punishment, taxation and political representation. Until recently these questions have not generally been associated with scientific research. However, they are foreshadowed even in the earliest reflections on the ethics of research involving human subjects. For example, during the 19th and early 20th centuries the burdens of serving as research subjects fell largely upon poor ward patients, while the benefits of improved medical care flowed primarily to private patients. Subsequently, the exploitation of unwilling prisoners as research subjects in Nazi concentration camps was condemned as a particularly flagrant injustice. In this country, in the 1940s, the Tuskegee syphilis study used disadvantaged, rural black men to study the untreated course of a disease that is by no means confined to that population. These subjects were deprived of demonstrably effective treatment in order not to interrupt the project, long after such treatment became generally available.

Against this historical background, it can be seen how conceptions of justice are relevant to research involving human subjects.

For example, the selection of research subjects needs to be scrutinized in order to determine whether some classes (e.g., welfare patients, particular racial and ethnic minorities, or persons confined to institutions) are being systematically selected simply because of their easy availability, their compromised position, or their manipulability, rather than for reasons directly related to the problem being studied. Finally, whenever research supported by public funds leads to the development of therapeutic devices and procedures, justice demands both that these not provide advantages only to those who can afford them and that such research should not unduly involve persons from groups unlikely to be among the beneficiaries of subsequent applications of the research.

Part C: Applications

C. Applications
Applications of the general principles to the conduct of research lead to consideration of the following requirements: informed consent, risk/benefit assessment, and the selection of subjects of research.

1. **Informed Consent**—Respect for persons requires that subjects, to the degree that they are capable, be given the opportunity to choose what shall or shall not happen to them. This opportunity is provided when adequate standards for informed consent are satisfied.

   While the importance of informed consent is unquestioned, controversy prevails over the nature and possibility of an informed consent. Nonetheless, there is widespread agreement that the consent process can be analyzed as containing three elements: information, comprehension and voluntariness.

   Information. Most codes of research establish specific items for disclosure intended to assure that subjects are given sufficient information. These items generally include: the research procedure, their purposes, risks and anticipated benefits, alternative procedures (where therapy is involved), and a statement offering the subject the opportunity to ask questions and to withdraw at any time from the research. Additional items have been proposed, including how subjects are selected, the person responsible for the research, etc.

   However, a simple listing of items does not answer the question of what the standard should be for judging how much and what sort of information should be provided. One standard frequently invoked in medical practice, namely the information commonly provided by practitioners in the field or in the locale, is inadequate since research takes place precisely when a common understanding does not exist. Another standard, currently popular in malpractice law, requires the practitioner to reveal the information that reasonable persons would wish to know in order to make a decision regarding their care. This, too, seems insufficient since the research subject, being in essence a volunteer, may wish to know considerably more about risks gratuitously undertaken than do patients who deliver themselves into the hand of a clinician for needed care. It may be that a standard of the "reasonable volunteer" should be proposed: the extent and nature of information should be such that persons, knowing that the procedure is neither necessary for their care nor perhaps fully understood, can decide whether they wish to participate in the furthering of knowledge. Even when some direct benefit to them is anticipated, the subjects should understand clearly the range of risk and the voluntary nature of participation.

A special problem of consent arises where informing subjects of some pertinent aspect of the research is likely to impair the validity of the research. In many cases, it is sufficient to indicate to subjects that they are being invited to participate in research of which some features will not be revealed until the research is concluded. In all cases of research involving incomplete disclosure, such research is justified only if it is clear that (1) incomplete disclosure is truly necessary to accomplish the goals of the research, (2) there are no undisclosed risks to subjects that are more than minimal, and (3) there is an adequate plan for debriefing subjects, when appropriate, and for dissemination of research results to them. Information about risks should never be withheld for the purpose of eliciting the cooperation of subjects, and truthful answers should always be given to direct questions about the research. Care should be taken to distinguish cases in which disclosure would destroy or invalidate the research from cases in which disclosure would simply inconvenience the investigator.

Comprehension. The manner and context in which information is conveyed is as important as the information itself. For example, presenting information in a disorganized and rapid fashion, allowing too little time for consideration or curtailing opportunities for questioning, all may adversely affect a subject's ability to make an informed choice.

Because the subject's ability to understand is a function of intelligence, rationality, maturity and language, it is necessary to adapt the presentation of the information to the subject's capacities. Investigators are responsible for ascertaining that the subject has comprehended the information. While there is always an obligation to ascertain that the information about risk to subjects is complete and adequately comprehended, when the risks are more serious, that obligation increases. On occasion, it may be suitable to give some oral or written tests of comprehension.

Special provision may need to be made when comprehension is severely limited—for example, by conditions of immaturity or mental disability. Each class of subjects that one might consider as incompetent (e.g., infants and young children, mentally disabled patients, the terminally ill and the comatose) should be considered on its own terms. Even for these persons, however, respect requires giving them the opportunity to choose to the extent they are able, whether or not to participate in research. The objections of these subjects to involvement should be honored, unless the research entails providing them a therapy unavailable elsewhere. Respect for persons also requires seeking the permission of other parties in order to protect the subjects from harm. Such persons are thus respected both by acknowledging their own wishes and by the use of third parties to protect them from harm.

The third parties chosen should be those who are most likely to understand the incompetent subject's situation and to act in that person's best interest. The person authorized to act on behalf of the subject should be given an opportunity to observe the research as it proceeds in order to be able to withdraw the subject from the research, if such action appears in the subject's best interest.

Voluntariness. An agreement to participate in research constitutes a valid consent only if voluntarily given. This element of informed consent requires conditions free of coercion and undue influence. Coercion occurs when an overt threat of harm is intentionally presented by one person to another in order to obtain compliance. Undue influence, by contrast, occurs through an offer of an excessive, unwarranted, inappropriate or improper reward or other overture in order to obtain compliance. Also, inducements that would ordinarily be acceptable may become undue influences if the subject is especially vulnerable.

Unjustifiable pressures usually occur when persons in positions of authority or commanding influence—especially where possible sanctions are involved—urge a course of action for a subject. A continuum of such influencing factors exists, however, and it is impossible to state precisely where justifiable persuasion ends and undue influence begins. But undue influence would include actions such as manipulating a person's choice through the controlling influence of a close relative and threatening to withdraw health services to which an individual would otherwise be entitled.

2. **Assessment of Risks and Benefits**—The assessment of risks and benefits requires a careful arrayal of relevant data, including, in some cases, alternative ways of obtaining the benefits sought in the research. Thus, the assessment presents both an opportunity and a responsibility to gather systematic and comprehensive information about proposed research. For the investigator, it is a means to examine whether the proposed research is properly designed. For a review committee, it is a method for determining whether the risks that will be presented to subjects are justified. For prospective subjects, the assessment will assist the determination whether or not to participate.

The Nature and Scope of Risks and Benefits. The requirement that research be justified on the basis of a favorable risk/benefit assessment bears a close relation to the principle of beneficence, just as the moral requirement that informed consent be obtained is derived primarily from the principle of respect for persons. The term "risk" refers to a possibility that harm may occur. However, when expressions such as "small risk" or "high risk" are used, they usually refer (often ambiguously) both to the chance (probability) of experiencing a harm and the severity (magnitude) of the envisioned harm.

The term "benefit" is used in the research context to refer to something of positive value related to health or welfare. Unlike, "risk," "benefit" is not a term that expresses probabilities. Risk is properly contrasted to probability of benefits, and benefits are properly contrasted with harms rather than risks of harm. Accordingly, so-called risk/benefit assessments are concerned with the probabilities and magnitudes of possible harm and anticipated benefits. Many kinds of possible harms and benefits need to be taken into account. There are, for example, risks of psychological harm, physical harm, legal harm, social harm and economic harm and the corresponding benefits. While the most likely types of harms to research subjects are those of psychological or physical pain or injury, other possible kinds should not be overlooked.

Risks and benefits of research may affect the individual subjects, the families of the individual subjects, and society at large (or special groups of subjects in society). Previous codes and Federal regulations have required that risks to subjects be outweighed by the sum of both the anticipated benefit to the subject, if any, and the anticipated bene-fit to society in the form of knowledge to be gained from the research. In balancing these different elements, the risks and benefits affecting the immediate research subject will normally carry special weight. On the other hand, interests other than those of the subject may on some occasions be sufficient by themselves to justify the risks involved in the research, so long as the subjects' rights have been protected. Beneficence thus requires that we protect against risk of harm to sub-jects and also that we be concerned about the loss of the substantial benefits that might be gained from research.

The Systematic Assessment of Risks and Benefits. It is com-monly said that benefits and risks must be "balanced" and shown to be "in a favorable ratio." The metaphorical character of these terms draws attention to the difficulty of making precise judgments. Only on rare occasions will quantitative techniques be available for the scrutiny of research protocols. However, the idea of systematic, nonarbitrary analysis of risks and benefits should be emulated inso-far as possible. This ideal requires those making decisions about the justifiability of research to be thorough in the accumulation and assessment of information about all aspects of the research, and to consider alternatives systematically. This procedure renders the assessment of research more rigorous and precise, while making com-munication between review board members and investigators less subject to misinterpretation, misinformation and conflicting judg-ments. Thus, there should first be a determination of the validity of the presuppositions of the research; then the nature, probability and magnitude of risk should be distinguished with as much clarity as possible. The method of ascertaining risks should be explicit, especially where there is no alternative to the use of such vague categories as small or slight risk. It should also be determined whether an investigator's estimates of the probability of harm or benefits are reasonable, as judged by known facts or other available studies.

Finally, assessment of the justifiability of research should reflect at least the following considerations: (i) Brutal or inhumane treatment of human subjects is never morally justified. (ii) Risks should be reduced to those necessary to achieve the research objective. It should be determined whether it is in fact necessary to use human subjects at all. Risk can perhaps never be entirely eliminated, but it can often be reduced by careful attention to alternative procedures. (iii) When research involves significant risk of serious impairment, review committees should be extraordinarily insistent on the justification of the risk (looking usually to the likelihood of benefit to the subject—or, in some rare cases, to the manifest voluntariness of the participation). (iv) When vulnerable populations are involved in research, the appropriateness of involving them should itself be demonstrated. A number of variables go into such judgments, including the nature and degree of risk, the condition of the particular population involved, and the nature and level of the anticipated benefits. (v) Relevant risks and benefits must be thoroughly arrayed in documents and procedures used in the informed consent process.

3. **Selection of Subjects**—Just as the principle of respect for persons finds expression in the requirements for consent, and the principle of beneficence in risk/benefit assessment, the principle of justice gives rise to moral requirements that there be fair procedures and outcomes in the selection of research subjects.

    Justice is relevant to the selection of subjects of research at two levels: the social and the individual. Individual justice in the selection of subjects would require that researchers exhibit fairness: thus, they should not offer potentially beneficial research only to some patients who are in their favor or select only "undesirable" persons for risky research. Social justice requires that distinction be drawn between classes of subjects that ought, and ought not, to participate in any particular kind of research, based on the ability of members of that class to bear burdens and on the appropriateness of placing further burdens on already burdened persons. Thus, it can be considered a matter of social justice that there is an order of preference in the selection of classes of subjects (e.g., adults before children) and that some classes of potential subjects (e.g., the institutionalized mentally infirm or prisoners) may be involved as research subjects, if at all, only on certain conditions.

Injustice may appear in the selection of subjects, even if individual subjects are selected fairly by investigators and treated fairly in the course of research. Thus injustice arises from social, racial, sexual and cultural biases institutionalized in society. Thus, even if individual researchers are treating their research subjects fairly, and even if Institutional Review Boards are taking care to assure that subjects are selected fairly within a particular institution, unjust social patterns may nevertheless appear in the overall distribution of the burdens and benefits of research. Although individual institutions or investigators may not be able to resolve a problem that is pervasive in their social setting, they can consider distributive justice in selecting research subjects.

Some populations, especially institutionalized ones, are already burdened in many ways by their infirmities and environments. When research is proposed that involves risks and does not include a therapeutic component, other less burdened classes of persons should be called upon first to accept these risks of research, except where the research is directly related to the specific conditions of the class involved. Also, even though public funds for research may often flow in the same directions as public funds for health care, it seems unfair that populations dependent on public health care constitute a pool of preferred research subjects if more advantaged populations are likely to be the recipients of the benefits.

One special instance of injustice results from the involvement of vulnerable subjects. Certain groups, such as racial minorities, the economically disadvantaged, the very sick, and the institutionalized may continually be sought as research subjects, owing to their ready availability in settings where research is conducted. Given their dependent status and their frequently compromised capacity for free consent, they should be protected against the danger of being involved in research solely for administrative convenience, or because they are easy to manipulate as a result of their illness or socioeconomic condition.

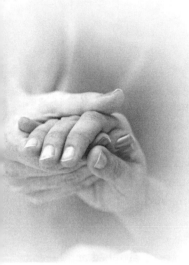

Appendix B

Nurses' Code of Ethics With Interpretive Statements

The nurse, in all professional relationships, practices with compassion and respect for the inherent dignity, worth and uniqueness of every individual, unrestricted by considerations of social or economic status, personal attributes, or the nature of health problems.

1.1 Respect for human dignity

A fundamental principle that underlies all nursing practice is respect for the inherent worth, dignity, and human rights of every individual. Nurses take into account the needs and values of all persons in all professional relationships.

1.2 Relationships to patients

The need for health care is universal, transcending all individual differences. The nurse establishes relationships and delivers nursing services with respect for human needs and values, and without prejudice. An individual's lifestyle, value system and religious beliefs should be considered in planning health care with and for each patient. Such consideration does not suggest that the nurse necessarily agrees with or condones certain individual choices, but that the nurse respects the patient as a person.

1.3 The nature of health problems

The nurse respects the worth, dignity and rights of all human beings irrespective of the nature of the health problem. The worth of the person is not affected by disease, disability, functional status, or proximity to death. This respect extends to all who require the services of the nurse for the promotion of health, the prevention of illness, the restoration of health, the alleviation of suffering, and the provision of supportive care to those who are dying.

The measures nurses take to care for the patient enable the patient to live with as much physical, emotional, social, and spiritual well-being as possible. Nursing care aims to maximize the values that the patient has treasured in life and extends supportive care to the family and significant others. Nursing care is directed toward meeting the comprehensive needs of patients and their families across the continuum of care. This is particularly vital in the care of patients and their families at the end of life to prevent and relieve the cascade of symptoms and suffering that are commonly associated with dying.

Nurses are leaders and vigilant advocates for the delivery of dignified and humane care. Nurses actively participate in assessing and assuring the responsible and appropriate use of interventions in order to minimize unwarranted or unwanted treatment and patient suffering. The acceptability and importance of carefully considered decisions regarding resuscitation status, withholding and withdrawing life-sustainings therapies, forgoing medically provided nutrition and hydration, aggressive pain and symptom management and advance directives are increasingly evident. The nurse should provide interventions to relieve pain and other symptoms in the dying patient even when those interventions entail risks of hastening death. However, nurses may not act with the sole intent of ending a patient's life even though such action may be motivated by compassion, respect for patient autonomy and quality of life considerations. Nurses have invaluable experience, knowledge, and insight into care at the end of life and should be actively involved in related research, education, practice, and policy development.

1.4 The right to self-determination
Respect for human dignity requires the recognition of specific patient rights, particularly, the right of self-determination. Self-determination, also known as autonomy, is the philosophical basis for informed consent in health care. Patients have the moral and legal right to determine what will be done with their own person; to be given accurate, complete, and understandable information in a manner that facilitates an informed judgment; to be assisted with weighing the benefits, burdens, and available options in their treatment, including the choice of no treatment; to accept, refuse, or terminate treatment without deceit, undue influence, duress, coercion, or penalty; and to be given necessary support throughout the decision-making and treatment process. Such support would include the opportunity to make decisions with family and significant others and the provision of advice and support from knowledgeable nurses and other health professionals. Patients

should be involved in planning their own health care to the extent they are able and choose to participate.

Each nurse has an obligation to be knowledgeable about the moral and legal rights of all patients to self-determination. The nurse preserves, protects, and supports those interests by assessing the patient's comprehension of both the information presented and the implications of decisions. In situations in which the patient lacks the capacity to make a decision, a designated surrogate decision-maker should be consulted. The role of the surrogate is to make decisions as the patient would, based upon the patient's previously expressed wishes and known values. In the absence of a designated surrogate decision-maker, decisions should be made in the best interests of the patient, considering the patient's personal values to the extent that they are known. The nurse supports patient self-determination by participating in discussions with surrogates, providing guidance and referral to other resources as necessary, and identifying and addressing problems in the decision-making process. Support of autonomy in the broadest sense also includes recognition that people of some cultures place less weight on individualism and choose to defer to family or community values in decision-making. Respect not just for the specific decision but also for the patient's method of decision-making is consistent with the principle of autonomy.

Individuals are interdependent members of the community. The nurse recognizes that there are situations in which the right to individual self-determination may be outweighed or limited by the rights, health and welfare of others, particularly in relation to public health considerations. Nonetheless, limitation of individual rights must always be considered a serious deviation from the standard of care, justified only when there are no less restrictive means available to preserve the rights of others and the demands of justice.

1.5 Relationships with colleagues and others
The principle of respect for persons extends to all individuals with whom the nurse interacts. The nurse maintains compassionate and caring relationships with colleagues and others with a commitment to the fair treatment of individuals, to integrity-preserving compromise, and to resolving conflict. Nurses function in many roles, including direct care provider, administrator, educator, researcher, and consultant. In each of these roles, the nurse treats colleagues, employees, assistants, and students with respect and compassion. This standard of conduct precludes any

and all prejudicial actions, any form of harassment or threatening behavior, or disregard for the effect of one's actions on others. The nurse values the distinctive contribution of individuals or groups, and collaborates to meet the shared goal of providing quality health services.

The nurse's primary commitment is to the patient, whether an individual, family, group or community.

2.1 Primacy of the patient's interests

The nurse's primary commitment is to the recipient of nursing and health care services—the patient—whether the recipient is an individual, a family, a group, or a community. Nursing holds a fundamental commitment to the uniqueness of the individual patient; therefore, any plan of care must reflect that uniqueness. The nurse strives to provide patients with opportunities to participate in planning care, assures that patients find the plans acceptable and supports the implementation of the plan. Addressing patient interests requires recognition of the patient's place in the family or other networks of relationship. When the patient's wishes are in conflict with others, the nurse seeks to help resolve the conflict. Where conflict persists, the nurse's commitment remains to the identified patient.

2.2 Conflict of interest for nurses

Nurses are frequently put in situations of conflict arising from competing loyalties in the workplace, including situations of conflicting expectations from patients, families, physicians, colleagues, and in many cases, health care organizations and health plans. Nurses must examine the conflicts arising between their own personal and professional values, the values and interests of others who are also responsible for patient care and health care decisions, as well as those of patients. Nurses strive to resolve such conflicts in ways that ensure patient safety, guard the patient's best interests and preserve the professional integrity of the nurse.

Situations created by changes in health care financing and delivery systems, such as incentive systems to decrease spending, pose new possibilities of conflict between economic self-interest and professional integrity. The use of bonuses, sanctions, and incentives tied to financial targets are examples of features of health care systems that may present such conflict. Conflicts of interest may arise in any domain of nursing activity including clinical practice, administration, education, or research. Advanced practice nurses who bill directly for services and nursing executives with budgetary responsibilities must be especially cognizant of the potential for conflicts of interest. Nurses should disclose to all relevant parties (e.g., patients, employers, colleagues) any perceived or actual conflict of interest and in some situations should withdraw from further participation. Nurses in all roles must seek to ensure that employment arrangements are just and fair and do not create an unreasonable conflict between patient care and direct personal gain.

2.3 Collaboration

Collaboration is not just cooperation, but it is the concerted effort of individuals and groups to attain a shared goal. In health care, that goal is to address the health needs of the patient and the public. The complexity of health care delivery systems requires a multi-disciplinary approach to the delivery of services that has the strong support and active participation of all the health professions. Within this context, nursing's unique contribution, scope of practice, and relationship with other health professions needs to be clearly articulated, represented, and preserved. By its very nature, collaboration requires mutual trust, recognition, and respect among the health care team, shared decision-making about patient care, and open dialogue among all parties who have an interest in and a concern for health outcomes. Nurses should work to assure that the relevant parties are involved and have a voice in decision-making about patient care issues. Nurses should see that the questions that need to be addressed are asked and that the information needed for informed decision-making is available and provided. Nurses should actively promote the collaborative multi-disciplinary planning required to ensure the availability and accessibility of quality health services to all persons who have needs for health care.

Intraprofessional collaboration within nursing is fundamental to effectively addressing the health needs of patients and the public. Nurses engaged in non-clinical roles, such as administration or research, while not providing direct care, nonetheless are collaborating in the provision of care through their influence and direction of those who do. Effective nursing care is accomplished through the interdependence of nurses in differing roles—those who teach the needed skills, set standards, manage the environment of care, or expand the boundaries of knowledge used by the profession. In this sense, nurses in all roles share a responsibility for the outcomes of nursing care.

2.4 Professional boundaries

When acting within one's role as a professional, the nurse recognizes and maintains boundaries that establish appropriate limits to relationships. While the nature of nursing work has an inherently personal component, nurse-patient relationships and nurse-colleague relationships have, as their foundation, the purpose of preventing illness, alleviating suffering, and protecting, promoting, and restoring the health of patients. In this way, nurse-patient and nurse-colleague relationships differ from those that are purely personal and unstructured, such as friendship. The intimate nature of nursing care, the involvement of nurses in important and sometimes highly stressful life events, and the mutual dependence of colleagues working in close concert all present the potential for blurring of limits to professional relationships. Maintaining authenticity and expressing oneself as an individual, while remaining within the bounds established by the purpose of the relationship, can be especially difficult in prolonged or long-term relationships. In all encounters, nurses are responsible for retaining their professional boundaries. When those professional boundaries are jeopardized, the nurse should seek assistance from peers or supervisors or take appropriate steps to remove her/himself from the situation.

The nurse promotes, advocates for, and strives to protect the health, safety, and rights of the patient.

3.1 Privacy
The nurse safeguards the patient's right to privacy. The need for health care does not justify unwanted intrusion into the patient's life. The nurse advocates for an environment that provides for sufficient physical privacy, including auditory privacy for discussions of a personal nature and policies and practices that protect the confidentiality of information.

3.2 Confidentiality
Associated with the right to privacy, the nurse has a duty to maintain confidentiality of all patient information. The patient's well-being could be jeopardized and the fundamental trust between patient and nurse destroyed by unnecessary access to data or by the inappropriate disclosure of identifiable patient information. The rights, well-being, and safety of the individual patient should be the primary factors in arriving at any professional judgment concerning the disposition of confidential information received from or about the patient, whether oral, written or electronic. The standard of nursing practice and the nurse's responsibility to provide quality care require that relevant data be shared with those members of the health care team who have a need to know. Only information pertinent to a patient's treatment and welfare is disclosed, and only to those directly involved with the patient's care.

Duties of confidentiality, however, are not absolute and may need to be modified in order to protect the patient, other innocent parties, and in circumstances of mandatory disclosure for public health reasons.

Information used for purposes of peer review, third-party payments, and other quality improvement or risk management mechanisms may be disclosed only under defined policies, mandates, or protocols. These written guidelines must assure that the rights, well-being, and safety of the patient are protected. In general, only that information directly relevant to a task or specific responsibility should be disclosed. When using electronic communication, special effort should be made to maintain data security.

3.3 Protection of participants in research

Stemming from the right to self-determination, each individual has the right to choose whether or not to participate in research. It is imperative that the patient or legally authorized surrogate receive sufficient information that is material to an informed decision, to comprehend that information, and to know how to discontinue participation in research without penalty. Necessary information to achieve an adequately informed consent includes the nature of participation, potential harms and benefits, and available alternatives to taking part in the research. Additionally, the patient should be informed of how the data will be protected. The patient has the right to refuse to participate in research or to withdraw at any time without fear of adverse consequences or reprisal.

Research should be conducted and directed only by qualified persons. Prior to implementation, all research should be approved by a qualified review board to ensure patient protection and the ethical integrity of the research. Nurses should be cognizant of the special concerns raised by research involving vulnerable groups, including children, prisoners, students, the elderly, and the poor. The nurse who participates in research in any capacity should be fully informed about both the subject's and the nurse's rights and obligations in the particular research study and in research in general. Nurses have the duty to question and, if necessary, to report and to refuse to participate in research they deem morally objectionable.

3.4 Standards and review mechanisms

Nursing is responsible and accountable for assuring that only those individuals who have demonstrated the knowledge, skill, practice experiences, commitment, and integrity essential to professional practice are allowed to enter into and continue to practice within the profession. Nurse educators have a responsibility to ensure that basic competencies are achieved and to promote a commitment to professional practice prior to entry of an individual into practice. Nurse administrators are responsible for assuring that the knowledge and skills of each nurse in the workplace are assessed prior to the assignment of responsibilities requiring preparation beyond basic academic programs.

The nurse has a responsibility to implement and maintain standards of professional nursing practice. The nurse should participate in planning, establishing, implementing, and evaluating review mechanisms designed to safeguard patients and nurses, such as peer review processes or committees, credentialing processes, quality improvement initiatives, and ethics committees. Nurse administrators must ensure that nurses have access to and inclusion on institutional ethics committees. Nurses must bring forward difficult issues related to patient care and/or institutional constraints upon ethical practice for discussion and review. The nurse acts to promote inclusion of appropriate others in all deliberations related to patient care.

Nurses should also be active participants in the development of policies and review mechanisms designed to promote patient safety, reduce the likelihood of errors, and address both environmental system factors and human factors that present increased risk to patients. In addition, when errors do occur, nurses are expected to follow institutional guidelines in reporting errors committed or observed to the appropriate supervisory personnel and for assuring responsible disclosure of errors to patients. Under no circumstances should the nurse participate in, or condone through silence, either an attempt to hide an error or a punitive response that serves only to fix blame rather than correct the conditions that led to the error.

3.5 Acting on questionable practice

The nurse's primary commitment is to the health, well-being, and safety of the patient across the life span and in all settings in which health care needs are addressed. As an advocate for the patient, the nurse must be alert to and take appropriate action regarding any instances of incompetent, unethical, illegal, or impaired practice by any member of the health care team or the health care system or any action on the part of others that places the rights or best interests of the patient in jeopardy. To function effectively in this role, nurses must be knowledgeable about the Code of Ethics, standards of practice of the profession, relevant federal, state and local laws and regulations, and the employing organization's policies and procedures.

When the nurse is aware of inappropriate or questionable practice in the provision or denial of health care, concern should be expressed to the person carrying out the questionable practice. Attention should be called to the possible detrimental affect upon the patient's well-being or best interests as well as the integrity of nursing practice. When factors in the health care delivery system or health care organization threaten the welfare of the patient, similar action should be directed to the responsible administrator. If indicated, the problem should be reported to an appropriate higher authority within the institution or agency, or to an appropriate external authority.

There should be established processes for reporting and handling incompetent, unethical, illegal, or impaired practice within the employment setting so that such reporting can go through official channels, thereby reducing the risk of reprisal against the reporting nurse. All nurses have a responsibility to assist those who identify potentially questionable practice. State nurses associations should be prepared to provide assistance and support in the development and evaluation of such processes and reporting procedures. When incompetent, unethical, illegal, or impaired practice is not corrected within the employment setting and continues to jeopardize patient well-being and safety, the problem should be reported to other appropriate authorities such as practice committees of the pertinent professional organizations, the legally constituted bodies concerned with licensing of specific categories of health workers and professional practitioners, or the regulatory agencies concerned with evaluating standards or practice. Some situations may warrant the concern and involvement of all such groups. Accurate reporting and factual documentation, and not merely opinion, undergird all such responsible actions. When a nurse chooses to engage in the act of responsible reporting about situations that are perceived as unethical, incompetent, illegal, or impaired, the professional organization has a responsibility to provide the nurse with support and assistance and to protect the practice of those nurses who choose to voice their concerns. Reporting unethical, illegal, incompetent, or impaired practices, even when done appropriately, may present substantial risks to the nurse; nevertheless, such risks do not eliminate the obligation to address serious threats to patient safety.

3.6 Addressing impaired practice
Nurses must be vigilant to protect the patient, the public, and the profession from potential harm when a colleague's practice, in any setting, appears to be impaired.

The nurse extends compassion and caring to colleagues who are in recovery from illness or when illness interferes with job performance. In a situation where a nurse suspects another's practice may be impaired, the nurse's duty is to take action designed both to protect patients and to assure that the impaired individual receives assistance in regaining optimal function. Such action should usually begin with consulting supervisory personnel and may also include confronting the individual in a supportive manner and with the assistance of others or helping the individual to access appropriate resources. Nurses are encouraged to follow guidelines outlined by the profession and policies of the employing organization to assist colleagues whose job performance may be adversely affected by mental or physical illness or by personal circumstances. Nurses in all roles should advocate for colleagues whose job performance may be impaired to ensure that they receive appropriate assistance, treatment and access to fair institutional and legal processes. This includes supporting the return to practice of the individual who has sought assistance and is ready to resume professional duties.

If impaired practice poses a threat or danger to self or others, regardless of whether the individual has sought help, the nurse must take action to report the individual to persons authorized to address the problem. Nurses who advocate for others whose job performance creates a risk for harm should be protected from negative consequences. Advocacy may be a difficult process and the nurse is advised to follow workplace policies. If workplace policies do not exist or are inappropriate—that is, they deny the nurse in question access to due legal process or demand resignation—the reporting nurse may obtain guidance from the professional association, state peer assistance programs, employee assistance program or a similar resource.

The nurse is responsible and accountable for individual nursing practice and determines the appropriate delegation of tasks consistent with the nurse's obligation to provide optimum patient care.

4.1 Acceptance of accountability and responsibility

Individual registered nurses bear primary responsibility for the nursing care that their patients receive and are individually accountable for their own practice. Nursing practice includes direct care activities, acts of delegation, and other responsibilities such as teaching, research, and administration. In each instance, the nurse retains accountability and responsibility for the quality of practice and for conformity with standards of care.

Nurses are faced with decisions in the context of the increased complexity and changing patterns in the delivery of health care. As the scope of nursing practice changes, the nurse must exercise judgment in accepting responsibilities, seeking consultation, and assigning activities to others who carry out nursing care. For example, some advanced practice nurses have the authority to issue prescription and treatment orders to be carried out by other nurses. These acts are not acts of delegation. Both the advanced practice nurse issuing the order and the nurse accepting the order are responsible for the judgments made and accountable for the actions taken.

4.2 Accountability for nursing judgment and action

Accountability means to be answerable to oneself and others for one's own actions. In order to be accountable, nurses act under a code of ethical conduct that is grounded in the moral principles of fidelity and respect for the dignity, worth, and self-determination of patients. Nurses are accountable for judgments made and actions taken in the course of nursing practice, irrespective of health care organizations' policies or providers' directives.

4.3 Responsibility for nursing judgment and action

Responsibility refers to the specific accountability or liability associated with the performance of duties of a particular role. Nurses accept or reject specific role demands based upon their education, knowledge, competence, and extent of experience. Nurses in administration, education, and research also have obligations to the recipients of nursing care. Although nurses in administration, education, and research have relationships with patients that are less direct, in assuming the responsibilities of a particular role, they share responsibility for the care provided by those whom they supervise and instruct. The nurse must not engage in practices prohibited by law or delegate activities to others that are prohibited by the practice acts of other health care providers.

Individual nurses are responsible for assessing their own competence. When the needs of the patient are beyond the qualifications and competencies of the nurse, consultation and collaboration must be sought from qualified nurses, other health professionals, or other appropriate sources. Educational resources should be sought by nurses and provided by institutions to maintain and advance the competence of nurses. Nurse educators act in collaboration with their students to assess the learning needs of the student, the effectiveness of the teaching program, the identification and utilization of appropriate resources, and the support needed for the learning process.

4.4 Delegation of nursing activities

Since the nurse is accountable for the quality of nursing care given to patients, nurses are accountable for the assignment of nursing responsibilities to other nurses and the delegation of nursing care activities to other health care workers. While delegation and assignment are used here in a generic moral sense, it is understood that individual states may have a particular legal definition of these terms.

The nurse must make reasonable efforts to assess individual competence when assigning selected components of nursing care to other health care workers. This assessment involves evaluating the knowledge, skills, and experience of the individual to whom the care is assigned, the complexity of the assigned tasks, and the health status of the patient. The nurse is also responsible for monitoring the activities of these individuals and evaluating the quality of the care provided. Nurses may not delegate responsibilities such as assessment and evaluation; they may delegate tasks. The nurse must not knowingly assign or delegate to any member of the nursing team a task for which that person is not prepared or qualified. Employer policies or directives do not relieve the nurse of responsibility for making judgments about the delegation and assignment of nursing care tasks.

Nurses functioning in management or administrative roles have a particular responsibility to provide an environment that supports and facilitates appropriate assignment and delegation. This includes providing appropriate orientation to staff, assisting less experienced nurses in developing necessary skills and competencies, and establishing policies and procedures that protect both the patient and nurse from the inappropriate assignment or delegation of nursing responsibilities, activities, or tasks.

Nurses functioning in educator or preceptor roles may have less direct relationships with patients. However, through assignment of nursing care activities to learners they share responsibility and accountability for the care provided. It is imperative that the knowledge and skills of the learner be sufficient to provide the assigned nursing care and that appropriate supervision be provided to protect both the patient and the learner.

The nurse owes the same duties to self as to others, including the responsi-
bility to preserve integrity and safety, to maintain competence, and to con-
tinue personal and professional growth.

5.1 Moral self-respect

Moral respect accords moral worth and dignity to all human beings irrespective of
their personal attributes or life situation. Such respect extends to oneself as well; the
same duties that we owe to others we owe to ourselves. Self-regarding duties refer
to a realm of duties that primarily concern oneself and include professional growth
and maintenance of competence, preservation of wholeness of character, and personal integrity.

5.2 Professional growth and maintenance of competence

Though it has consequences for others, maintenance of competence and ongoing
professional growth involves the control of one's own conduct in a way that is primarily self-regarding. Competence affects one's self-respect, self-esteem, professional
status, and the meaningfulness of work. In all nursing roles, evaluation of one's own
performance, coupled with peer review, is a means by which nursing practice can be
held to the highest standards. Each nurse is responsible for participating in the
development of criteria for evaluation of practice and for using those criteria in peer
and self-assessment.

Continual professional growth, particularly in knowledge and skill, requires a commitment to lifelong learning. Such learning includes, but is not limited to, continuing education, networking with professional colleagues, self-study, professional
reading, certification, and seeking advanced degrees. Nurses are required to have
knowledge relevant to the current scope and standards of nursing practice, changing issues, concerns, controversies, and ethics. Where the care required is outside
the competencies of the individual nurse, consultation should be sought or the
patient should be referred to others for appropriate care.

5.3 Wholeness of character

Nurse have both personal and professional identities that are neither entirely separate, nor entirely merged, but are integrated. In the process of becoming a professional, the nurse embraces the values of the profession, integrating them with
personal values. Duties to self involve an authentic expression of one's own moral
point-of-view in practice. Sound ethical decision-making requires the respectful

and open exchange of views between and among all individuals with relevant interests. In a community of moral discourse, no one person's view should automatically take precedence over that of another. Thus the nurse has a responsibility to express moral perspectives, even when they differ from those of others, and even when they might not prevail.

This wholeness of character encompasses relationships with patients. In situations where the patient requests a personal opinion from the nurse, the nurse is generally free to express an informed personal opinion as long as this preserves the voluntariness of the patient and maintains appropriate professional and moral boundaries. It is essential to be aware of the potential for undue influence attached to the nurse's professional role. Assisting patients to clarify their own values in reaching informed decisions may be helpful in avoiding unintended persuasion. In situations where nurses' responsibilities include care for those whose personal attributes, condition, lifestyle, or situation is stigmatized by the community and are personally unacceptable, the nurse still renders respectful and skilled care.

5.4 Preservation of integrity

Integrity is an aspect of wholeness of character and is primarily a self-concern of the individual nurse. An economically constrained health care environment presents the nurse with particularly troubling threats to integrity. Threats to integrity may include a request to deceive a patient, to withhold information, or to falsify records, as well as verbal abuse from patients or coworkers. Threats to integrity also may include an expectation that the nurse will act in a way that is inconsistent with the values or ethics of the profession, or more specifically a request that is in direct violation of the Code of Ethics. Nurses have a duty to remain consistent with both their personal and professional values and to accept compromise only to the degree that it remains an integrity-preserving compromise. An integrity-preserving compromise does not jeopardize the dignity or well-being of the nurse or others. Integrity-preserving compromise can be difficult to achieve, but is more likely to be accomplished in situations where there is an open forum for moral discourse and an atmosphere of mutual respect and regard.

Where nurses are placed in situations of compromise that exceed acceptable moral limits or involve violations of the moral standards of the profession, whether in direct patient care or in any other forms of nursing practice, they may express their conscientious objection to participation. Where a particular treatment, intervention, activity, or practice is morally objectionable to the nurse, whether intrinsically so or because it is inappropriate for the specific patient, or where it may jeopardize both patients and nursing practice, the nurse is justified in refusing to participate on moral grounds. Such grounds exclude personal preference, prejudice, convenience, or arbitrariness. Conscientious objection may not insulate the nurse against formal or informal penalty. The nurse who decides not to take part on the grounds of conscientious objection must communicate this decision in appropriate ways. Whenever possible, such a refusal should be made known in advance and in time for alternate arrangements to be made for patient care. The nurse is obliged to provide for the patient's safety, to avoid patient abandonment, and to withdraw only when assured that alternative sources of nursing care are available to the patient.

Where patterns of institutional behavior or professional practice compromise the integrity of all its nurses, nurses should express their concern or conscientious objection collectively to the appropriate body or committee. In addition, they should express their concern, resist, and seek to bring about a change in those persistent activities or expectations in the practice setting that are morally objectionable to nurses and jeopardize either patient or nurse well-being.

The nurse participates in establishing, maintaining, and improving health care environments and conditions of employment conducive to the provision of quality health care and consistent with the values of the profession through individual and collective action.

6.1 Influence of the environment on moral virtues and values
Virtues are habits of character that predispose persons to meet their moral obligations; that is, to do what is right. Excellences are habits of character that predispose a person to do a particular job or task well. Virtues such as wisdom, honesty, and courage are habits or attributes of the morally good person. Excellences such as compassion, patience, and skill are habits of character of the morally good nurse. For the nurse, virtues and excellences are those habits that affirm and promote the values of human dignity, well-being, respect, health, independence, and other values central to nursing. Both virtues and excellences, as aspects of moral character, can be either nurtured by the environment in which the nurse practices or they can be diminished or thwarted. All nurses have a responsibility to create, maintain, and contribute to environments that support the growth of virtues and excellences and enable nurses to fulfill their ethical obligations.

6.2 Influence of the environment on ethical obligations

All nurses, regardless of role, have a responsibility to create, maintain, and contribute to environments of practice that support nurses in fulfilling their ethical obligations. Environments of practice include observable features, such as working conditions, and written policies and procedures setting out expectations for nurses, as well as less tangible characteristics such as informal peer norms. Organizational structures, role descriptions, health and safety initiatives, grievance mechanisms, ethics committees, compensation systems, and disciplinary procedures all contribute to environments that can either present barriers or foster ethical practice and professional fulfillment. Environments in which employees are provided fair hearing of grievances, are supported in practicing according to standards of care, and are justly treated allow for the realization of the values of the profession and are consistent with sound nursing practice.

6.3 Responsibility for the health care environment

The nurse is responsible for contributing to a moral environment that encourages respectful interactions with colleagues, support of peers, and identification of issues that need to be addressed. Nurse administrators have a particular responsibility to assure that employees are treated fairly and that nurses are involved in decisions related to their practice and working conditions. Acquiescing and accepting unsafe or inappropriate practices, even if the individual does not participate in the specific practice, is equivalent to condoning unsafe practice. Nurses should not remain employed in facilities that routinely violate patient rights or require nurses to severely and repeatedly compromise standards of practice or personal morality.

As with concerns about patient care, nurses should address concerns about the health care environment through appropriate channels. Organizational changes are difficult to accomplish and may require persistent efforts over time. Toward this end, nurses may participate in collective action such as collective bargaining or workplace advocacy, preferably through a professional association such as the state nurses association, in order to address the terms and conditions of employment. Agreements reached through such action must be consistent with the profession's standards of practice, the state law regulating practice, and the Code of Ethics for Nursing. Conditions of employment must contribute to the moral environment, the provision of quality patient care, and the professional satisfaction for nurses.

The professional association also serves as an advocate for the nurse by seeking to secure just compensation and humane working conditions for nurses. To accomplish this, the professional association may engage in collective bargaining on behalf of nurses. While seeking to assure just economic and general welfare for nurses, collective bargaining, nonetheless, seeks to keep the interests of both nurses and patients in balance.

The nurse participates in the advancement of the profession through contributions to practice, education, administration, and knowledge development.

7.1 Advancing the profession through active involvement in nursing and in health care policy

Nurses should advance their profession by contributing in some way to the leadership, activities, and the viability of their professional organizations. Nurses can also advance the profession by serving in leadership or mentorship roles or on committees within their places of employment. Nurses who are self-employed can advance the profession by serving as role models for professional integrity. Nurses can also advance the profession through participation in civic activities related to health care or through local, state, national, or international initiatives. Nurse educators have a specific responsibility to enhance students' commitment to professional and civic values. Nurse administrators have a responsibility to foster an employment environment that facilitates nurses' ethical integrity and professionalism, and nurse researchers are responsible for active contribution to the body of knowledge supporting and advancing nursing practice.

7.2 Advancing the profession by developing, maintaining, and implementing professional standards in clinical, administrative, and educational practice

Standards and guidelines reflect the practice of nursing grounded in ethical commitments and a body of knowledge. Professional standards and guidelines for nurses must be developed by nurses and reflect nursing's responsibility to society. It is the responsibility of nurses to identify their own scope of practice as permitted by professional practice standards and guidelines, by state and federal laws, by relevant societal values, and by the Code of Ethics.

The nurse as administrator or manager must establish, maintain, and promote conditions of employment that enable nurses within that organization or community setting to practice in accord with accepted standards of nursing practice and provide a nursing and health care work environment that meets the standards and guidelines of nursing practice. Professional autonomy and self regulation in the control of conditions of practice are necessary for implementing nursing standards and guidelines and assuring quality care for those whom nursing serves.

The nurse educator is responsible for promoting and maintaining optimum standards of both nursing education and of nursing practice in any settings where planned learning activities occur. Nurse educators must also ensure that only those students who possess the knowledge, skills, and competencies that are essential to nursing graduate from their nursing programs.

7.3 Advancing the profession through knowledge development, dissemination, and application to practice

The nursing profession should engage in scholarly inquiry to identify, evaluate, refine, and expand the body of knowledge that forms the foundation of its discipline and practice. In addition, nursing knowledge is derived from the sciences and from the humanities. Ongoing scholarly activities are essential to fulfilling a profession's obligations to society. All nurses working alone or in collaboration with others can participate in the advancement of the profession through the development, evaluation, dissemination, and application of knowledge in practice. However, an organizational climate and infrastructure conducive to scholarly inquiry must be valued and implemented for this to occur.

The nurse collaborates with other health professionals and the public in promoting community, national, and international efforts to meet health needs.

8.1 Health needs and concerns

The nursing profession is committed to promoting the health, welfare, and safety of all people. The nurse has a responsibility to be aware not only of specific health needs of individual patients but also of broader health concerns such as world hunger, environmental pollution, lack of access to health care, violation of human rights, and inequitable distribution of nursing and health care resources. The availability and accessibility of high quality health services to all people require both interdisciplinary planning and collaborative partnerships among health professionals and others at the community, national, and international levels.

8.2 Responsibilities to the public

Nurses, individually and collectively, have a responsibility to be knowledgeable about the health status of the community and existing threats to health and safety. Through support of and participation in community organizations and groups, the nurse assists in efforts to educate the public, facilitates informed choice, identifies conditions and circumstances that contribute to illness, injury and disease, fosters healthy life styles, and participates in institutional and legislative efforts to promote health and meet national health objectives. In addition, the nurse supports initiatives to address barriers to health, such as poverty, homelessness, unsafe living conditions, abuse and violence, and lack of access to health services.

The nurse also recognizes that health care is provided to culturally diverse populations in this country and in all parts of the world. In providing care, the nurse should avoid imposition of the nurse's own cultural values upon others. The nurse should affirm human dignity and show respect for the values and practices associated with different cultures and use approaches to care that reflect awareness and sensitivity.

The profession of nursing, as represented by associations and their members, is responsible for articulating nursing values, for maintaining the integrity of the profession and its practice, and for shaping social policy.

9.1 Assertion of values

It is the responsibility of a professional association to communicate and affirm the values of the profession to its members. It is essential that the professional organization encourages discourse that supports critical self-reflection and evaluation within the profession. The organization also communicates to the public the values that nursing considers central to social change that will enhance health.

9.2 The profession carries out its collective responsibility through professional associations

The nursing profession continues to develop ways to clarify nursing's accountability to society. The contract between the profession and society is made explicit through such mechanisms as (a) the Code of Ethics for Nurses, (b) the standards of nursing practice, (c) the ongoing development of nursing knowledge derived from nursing theory, scholarship, and research in order to guide nursing actions, (d) educational requirements for practice, (e) certification, and (f) mechanisms for evaluating the effectiveness of professional nursing actions.

9.3 Intraprofessional integrity

A professional association is responsible for expressing the values and ethics of the profession and also for encouraging the professional organization and its members to function in accord with those values and ethics. Thus, one of its fundamental responsibilities is to promote awareness of and adherence to the Code of Ethics and to critique the activities and ends of the professional association itself. Values and ethics influence the power structures of the association in guiding, correcting, and directing its activities. Legitimate concerns for the self-interest of the association and the profession are balanced by a commitment to the social goods that are sought. Through critical self-reflection and self-evaluation, associations must foster change within themselves, seeking to move the professional community toward its stated ideals.

9.4 Social reform

Nurses can work individually as citizens or collectively through political action to bring about social change. It is the responsibility of a professional nursing association to speak for nurses collectively in shaping and reshaping health care within our nation, specifically in areas of health care policy and legislation that affect accessibility, quality, and the cost of health care. Here, the professional association maintains vigilance and takes action to influence legislators, reimbursement agencies, nursing organizations, and other health professions. In these activities, health is understood as being broader than delivery and reimbursement systems, but extending to health-related sociocultural issues such as violation of human rights, homelessness, hunger, violence, and the stigma of illness.

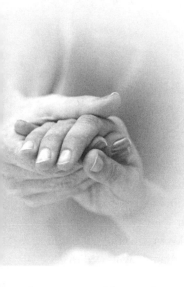

Appendix C

The Patient Care Partnership: Understanding Expectations, Rights and Responsibilities

When you need hospital care, your doctor and the nurses and other professionals at our hospital are committed to working with you and your family to meet your health care needs. Our dedicated doctors and staff serve the community in all its ethnic, religious and economic diversity. Our goal is for you and your family to have the same care and attention we would want for our families and ourselves.

The sections explain some of the basics about how you can expect to be treated during your hospital stay. They also cover what we will need from you to care for you better. If you have questions at any time, please ask them. Unasked or unanswered questions can add to the stress of being in the hospital. Your comfort and confidence in your care are very important to us.

What to Expect During Your Hospital Stay

- **High quality hospital care.** Our first priority is to provide you the care you need, when you need it, with skill, compassion, and respect. Tell your caregivers if you have concerns about your care or if you have pain. You have the right to know the identity of doctors, nurses and others involved in your care, and you have the right to know when they are students, residents or other trainees.

- **A clean and safe environment.** Our hospital works hard to keep you safe. We use special policies and procedures to avoid mistakes in your care and keep you free from abuse or neglect. If anything unexpected and significant happens during your hospital stay, you will be told what happened, and any resulting changes in your care will be discussed with you.

185

- **Involvement in your care.** You and your doctor often make decisions
  about your care before you go to the hospital. Other times, especially in
  emergencies, those decisions are made during your hospital stay. When
  decision-making takes place, it should include: *Discussing your medical
  condition and information about medically appropriate treatment
  choices:* To make informed decisions with your doctor, you need to
  understand: the benefits and risks of each treatment, whether your
  treatment is experimental or part of a research study, what you can rea-
  sonably expect from your treatment and any long-term effects it might
  have on your quality of life, what you and your family will need to do
  after you leave the hospital, the financial consequences of using uncovered services or out-of-network providers. Please tell your caregivers if
  you need more information about treatment choices. *Discussing your
  treatment plan:* When you enter the hospital, you sign a general consent to treatment. In some cases, such as surgery or experimental treatment, you may be asked to confirm in writing that you understand
  what is planned and agree to it. This process protects your right to
  consent to or refuse a treatment. Your doctor will explain the medical
  consequences of refusing recommended treatment. It also protects your
  right to decide if you want to participate in a research study. *Getting
  information from you:*. Your caregivers need complete and correct information about your health and coverage so that they can make good
  decisions about your care. That includes: Past illnesses, surgeries or hospital stays, past allergic reactions, any medicines or dietary supplements
  (such as vitamins and herbs) that you are taking, any network or admis-
  sion requirements under your health plan. *Understanding your health
  care goals and values:* You may have health care goals and values or spiritual beliefs that are important to your well-being. They will be taken
  into account as much as possible throughout your hospital stay. Make
  sure your doctor, your family and your care team know your wishes.
  Understanding who should make decisions when you cannot: If you
  have signed a health care power of attorney stating who should speak
  for you if you become unable to make health care decisions for yourself,
  or a "living will" or "advance directive" that states your wishes about
  end-of-life care; give copies to your doctor, your family and your care
  team; if you or your family need help making difficult decisions,
  counselors, chaplains and others are available to help.

- **Protection of your privacy.** We respect the confidentiality of your relationship with your doctor and other caregivers, and the sensitive information about your health and health care that are part of that relationship. State and federal laws and hospital operating policies protect the privacy of your medical information. You will receive a Notice of Privacy Practices that describes the ways that we use, disclose and safeguard patient information and that explains how you can obtain a copy of information from our records about your care.

- **Preparing you and your family for when you leave the hospital.** Your doctor works with hospital staff and professionals in your community. You and your family also play an important role in your care. The success of your treatment often depends on your efforts to follow medication, diet and therapy plans. Your family may need to help care for you at home.

    You can expect us to help you identify sources of follow-up care and to let you know if our hospital has a financial interest in any referrals. As long as you agree that we can share information about your care with them, we will coordinate our activities with your caregivers outside the hospital. You can also expect to receive information and, where possible, training about the self-care you will need when you go home.

- **Help with your bill and filing insurance claims.** Our staff will file claims for you with health care insurers or other programs such as Medicare and Medicaid. They also will help your doctor with needed documentation. Hospital bills and insurance coverage are often confusing. If you have questions about your bill, contact our business office. If you need help understanding your insurance coverage or health plan, start with your insurance company or health benefits manager. If you do not have health coverage, we will try to help you and your family find financial help or make other arrangements. We need your help with collecting needed information and other requirements to obtain coverage or assistance.

    While you are here, you will receive more detailed notices about some of the rights you have as a hospital patient and how to exercise them. We are always interested in improving. [...]

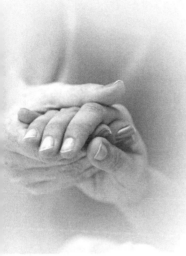

Appendix D

The American Nurses Association's Bill of Rights for Registered Nurses

Registered nurses promote and restore health, prevent illness and protect the people entrusted to their care. They work to alleviate the suffering experienced by individuals, families, groups and communities. In so doing, nurses provide services that maintain respect for human dignity and embrace the uniqueness of each patient and the nature of his or her health problems, without restriction with regard to social or economic status. To maximize the contributions nurses make to society, it is necessary to protect the dignity and autonomy of nurses in the workplace. To that end, the following rights must be afforded:

1. Nurses have the right to practice in a manner that fulfills their obligations to society and to those who receive nursing care.

2. Nurses have the right to practice in environments that allow them to act in accordance with professional standards and legally authorized scopes of practice.

3. Nurses have the right to a work environment that supports and facilitates ethical practice, in accordance with the Code of Ethics for Nurses and its interpretive statements.

4. Nurses have the right to freely and openly advocate for themselves and their patients, without fear of retribution.

5. Nurses have the right to fair compensation for their work, consistent with their knowledge, experience and professional responsibilities.

6. Nurses have the right to a work environment that is safe for themselves and their patients.

7. Nurses have the right to negotiate the conditions of their employment, either as individuals or collectively, in all practice settings.

Disclaimer: The American Nurses Association (ANA) is a national professional association. ANA policies reflect the thinking of the nursing profession on various issues and should be reviewed in conjunction with state association policies and state board of nursing policies and practices. State law, rules and regulation govern nursing. The ANA's "Bill of Rights for Registered Nurses" contains policy statements and does not necessarily reflect rights embodied in state and federal law. ANA policies may be used by the state to interpret or provide guidance on the profession's position on nursing.

Permissions

Reprinted with permission from American Nurses Association. *ANA's Bill of Rights for Registered Nurses*, ©2001 Nursesbooks.org, Silver Spring, Md.

This Bill of Rights was adopted by the ANA Board of Directors on June 26, 2001.

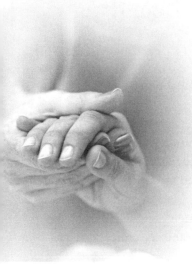

Appendix E

Nursing's Social Policy Statement

Introduction

"Nursing is the pivotal health care profession, highly valued for its specialized knowledge, skill and caring in improving the health status of the public and ensuring safe, effective, quality care. The profession mirrors the diverse population it serves and provides leadership to create positive changes in health policy and delivery systems. Individuals choose nursing as a career, and remain in the profession, because of the opportunities for personal and professional growth, supportive work environments and compensation commensurate with roles and responsibilities.[1]

The Social Context of Nursing

Nursing's Social Policy Statement, Second Edition expresses the social contract between society and the profession of nursing. Registered nurses and others can use this document as a framework for understanding professional nursing's relationship with society and its obligation to those who receive professional nursing care. It includes a definition of professional nursing, descriptions of professional nursing and its knowledge base, and brief descriptions of the scope of professional nursing practice and the methods by which the profession is regulated. These concepts underlie the practice of professional nursing, provide direction for clinicians, educators, administrators, and scientists within professional nursing, and inform other health care professionals, public policymakers, and funding bodies about professional nursing's contribution to health care.

This statement is derived from the 1980 landmark document, *Nursing: A Social Policy Statement,*[2] and *Nursing's Social Policy Statement,*[3] published in 1995. These documents provided the profession's earlier descriptions of its social responsibility and professional nursing's roles in the American health care system. The current document presents the practice of professional nursing as it has evolved, and provides direction for the future.

Professional nursing, like other professions, is an essential part of the society from which it grew and within which it continues to evolve. Professional nursing is dynamic, rather than static, reflecting the changing nature of societal needs. Professional nursing can be said to be owned by society, in the sense that "a profession acquires recognition, relevance, and even meaning in terms of its relationship to that society, its culture and institutions, and its other members."[4] This social contract between the broader society and its professions has been expressed as follows:

> Societies (and often vested Interests within them)...determine, in accord with their different technological and economic levels of development and their socioeconomic, political and cultural conditions and values, what professional skills and knowledge they most need or desire...Logically, then, the professions open to individuals in any particular society are the property not of the individual but of the society. What individuals acquire through training is professional knowledge and skill, not a profession or even part ownership of one.[5]

The authority for the practice of professional nursing is based on a social contract that acknowledges professional rights and responsibilities as well as mechanisms for public accountability.

> Society grants the professions authority over functions vital to itself and permits them considerable autonomy in the conduct of their affairs. In return, the professions are expected to act responsibly, always mindful of the public trust. Self-regulation to assure quality in performance is at the heart of this relationship. It is the authentic hallmark of a mature profession.[6]

To maximize the contributions nurses make to society, it is necessary to protect the dignity and autonomy of nurses in the workplace. To that end, the American Nurses Association has adopted the *Bill of Rights for Registered Nurses.*[7]

Values and Assumptions of Nursing's Social Contract

The following values and assumptions undergird professional nursing's contract with society:

- Humans manifest an essential unity of mind, body, and spirit.
- Human experience is contextually and culturally defined.
- Health and illness are human experiences. The presence of illness does not preclude health nor does optimal health preclude illness.
- The relationship between nurse and patient involves participation of both in the process of care.
- The interaction between nurse and patient occurs within the context of the values and beliefs of the patient and the nurse.
- Public policy and the health care delivery system influence the health and well-being of society and professional nursing.

These values and assumptions apply whether the recipient of professional nursing care is an individual, family, group, community, or population.

Definition of Nursing

Definitions of nursing have evolved to acknowledge six essential features of professional nursing:

- provision of a caring relationship that facilitates health and healing,
- attention to the range of human experiences and responses to health and illness within the physical and social environments,
- integration of objective data with knowledge gained from an appreciation of the patient or group's subjective experience,
- application of scientific knowledge to the processes of diagnosis and treatment through the use of judgment and critical thinking,
- advancement of professional nursing knowledge through scholarly inquiry, and
- influence on social and public policy to promote social justice.

In her *Notes on Nursing: What It Is and What It Is Not*, published in 1859, Florence Nightingale defined nursing as having "charge of the personal health of somebody ... and what nursing has to do ... is to put the patient in the best condition for nature to act upon him."[8]

A century later, Virginia Henderson defined the purpose of nursing as "to assist the individual, sick or well, in the performance of those activities contributing to health or its recovery (or to a peaceful death) that he would perform unaided if he had the necessary strength, will or knowledge. And to do this in such a way as to help him gain independence as rapidly as possible."[9]

In the 1980 *Nursing: A Social Policy Statement*, nursing was defined as "the diagnosis and treatment of human responses to actual or potential health problems."[10]

A broader definition is consistent with professional nursing's commitment to meeting societal needs, and permits the profession and its practitioners to adapt to the ongoing changes in healthcare environments, practice expectations, and the profession itself. The evolution of nursing practice leads to the following definition of professional nursing:

> Nursing is the protection, promotion, and optimization of health and abilities, prevention of illness and injury, alleviation of suffering through the diagnosis and treatment of human response, and advocacy in the care of individuals, families, communities, and populations.[11]

Moreover, nursing addresses the organizational, social, economic, legal, and political factors within the health care system and society. These and other factors affect the cost, access to, and quality of health care and the vitality of the nursing profession. This is accomplished through a variety of means.

Knowledge Base for Nursing Practice

Nursing is a profession and a scientific discipline. The knowledge base for professional nursing practice includes nursing science, philosophy, and ethics, as well as physical, economic, biomedical, behavioral, and social sciences. To refine and expand the knowledge base and science of the discipline, nurses generate and use theories and research findings that are selected on the basis of their fit with professional nursing's values of health and health care, as well as their relevance to professional nursing practice.

Nurses are concerned with human experiences and responses across the lifespan. Nurses partner with individuals, families, communities, and populations to address issues such as:

- promotion of health and safety;
- care and self-care processes;
- physical, emotional, and spiritual comfort, discomfort, and pain;

- adaptation to physiologic and pathophysiologic processes;
- emotions related to experiences of birth, growth and development, health, illness, disease, and death;
- meanings ascribed to health and illness;
- decision-making and ability to make choices;
- relationships, role performance, and change processes within relationships;
- social policies and their effects on the health of individuals, families, and communities;
- health care systems and their relationships with access to and quality of health care; and
- the environment and the prevention of disease.

Nurses use their theoretical and evidence-based knowledge of these phenomena in collaborating with patients to assess, plan, implement, and evaluate care. Nursing interventions are intended to produce beneficial effects and contribute to quality outcomes. Nurses evaluate the effectiveness of their care in relation to identified outcomes and use evidence to improve care.

Scope of Nursing Practice

Professional nursing has one scope of practice, which encompasses the range of activities from those of the beginning registered nurse through the advanced level. While a single scope of professional nursing practice exists, the depth and breadth to which individual nurses engage in the total scope of professional nursing practice is dependent on their educational preparation, their experience, their role, and the nature of the patient population they serve.

Further, all nurses are responsible for practicing in accordance with recognized standards of professional nursing practice and professional performance. The level of application of standards varies with the education, experience, and skills of the individual nurse. Since 1965, ANA has consistently affirmed the baccalaureate degree in nursing as the preferred educational requirement for entry into professional nursing practice.[12] Each nurse remains accountable for the quality of care within his or her scope of nursing practice.

Professional nursing's scope of practice is dynamic and continually evolving. It has a flexible boundary that is responsive to the changing needs of society and the expanding knowledge base of its theoretical and scientific domains. This scope of practice thus overlaps those of other professions involved in health care. The boundaries of each profession are constantly changing, and members of various professions cooperate by sharing knowledge, techniques, and ideas about how to deliver quality health care. Collaboration among health care professionals involves recognition of the expertise of others within and outside the profession, and referral to those other providers when appropriate. Collaboration also involves some shared functions and a common focus on the same overall mission.

Nurses provide care for patients in a variety of settings. Nurses may initiate treatments or carry out interventions initiated by other authorized health care providers. Nurses are coordinators of care as well as caregivers.

Nursing practice includes, but is not limited to, initiating and maintaining comfort measures, promoting and supporting human functions and responses, establishing an environment conducive to well-being, providing health counseling and teaching, and collaborating on certain aspects of the health regimen. This practice is based on understanding the human condition across the life span and the relationship of the individual within the environment.

Nursing care is provided and directed by registered nurses and advanced practice registered nurses. All registered nurses are educated in the art and science of nursing with the goal of helping patients to attain, maintain, and restore health, or to experience a dignified death. Registered nurses and advanced practice registered nurses may also develop expertise in a particular specialty.

Specialization in Nursing

Specialization involves focusing on a part of the whole field of professional nursing. The American Nurses Association and specialty nursing organizations delineate the components of professional nursing practice that are essential for any particular specialty. Registered nurses may seek certification in a variety of specialized areas of nursing practice.

Advanced Practice Registered Nurses

Advanced practice registered nurses (that is, nurse practitioners, certified registered nurse anesthetists, certified nurse-midwives, and clinical nurse specialists) practice from both *expanded* and *specialized* knowledge and skills.

- *Expansion* refers to the acquisition of new practice knowledge and skills, including the knowledge and skills that authorize role autonomy within areas of practice that may overlap traditional boundaries of medical practice.

- *Specialization* is concentrating or delimiting one's focus to part of the whole field of professional nursing (such as ambulatory care, pediatric, maternal-child, psychiatric, palliative care, or oncology nursing).

Advanced practice is characterized by the integration and application of a broad range of theoretical and evidence-based knowledge that occurs as a part of graduate nursing education. Advanced practice registered nurses hold master's or doctoral degrees and are licensed, certified, and/or approved to practice in their roles.

Additional Advanced Roles

Continuation of the profession of nursing is also dependent on the education of nurses, appropriate organization of nursing services, continued expansion of nursing knowledge, and the development and adoption of policies consistent with values and assumptions that underlie the scope of professional nursing practice. Registered nurses may practice in such advanced roles as nurse educator, nurse administrator, nurse researcher, and nurse policy analyst. These advanced roles require specific additional knowledge and skills at the graduate level. Generally, those practicing in these roles hold master's or doctoral degrees.

Further details on the scope of professional nursing practice, specifics describing the *who, what, where, when, why,* and *how* of both specialized and advanced areas of nursing practice, are found in the current version of *Nursing: Scope and Standards of Practice.*[13]

The Regulation of Nursing Practice

Professional nursing, like other professions, is accountable for ensuring that its members act in the public interest in the course of providing the unique service society has entrusted to them. The processes by which the profession does this include self-regulation, professional regulation, and legal regulation.

Self-Regulation

Self-regulation involves personal accountability for the knowledge base for professional practice. Nurses develop and maintain current knowledge, skills, and abilities through formal and continuing education. Where appropriate, nurses hold certification in their area of practice to demonstrate this accountability.

Nurses also regulate themselves as individuals through peer review of their practice. Continuous performance improvement fosters the refinement of knowledge, skills, and clinical decision-making processes at all levels and in all areas of professional nursing practice. As expressed in the profession's code of ethics, peer review is one mechanism by which nurses are held accountable for practice.

As noted in Provision 3.4 (Standards and Review Mechanisms) of *Code of Ethics for Nurses with Interpretive Statements*,[14] nurses should also be active participants in the development of policies and review mechanisms designed to promote patient safety, reduce the likelihood of errors, and address both environmental system factors and human factors that present increased risk to patients. In addition, when errors do occur, nurses are expected to follow established guidelines in reporting errors committed or observed.

Professional Regulation

Professional nursing defines its practice base, provides for research and development of that practice base, establishes a system for nursing education, establishes the structures through which nursing services will be delivered, and provides quality review mechanisms such as a code of ethics, standards of practice, structures for peer review, and a system of credentialing.

Professional regulation of nursing practice begins with the profession's definition of nursing and the scope of professional nursing practice. Professional standards are then derived from the scope of professional nursing practice.

Certification is a judgment of competence made by nurses who are themselves practicing within the area of specialization. Several credentialing boards are associated with the American Nurses Association and with specialty nursing organizations. These boards develop and implement certification examinations and procedures for nurses who wish to have their specialty practice knowledge recognized by the profession and the public. One component of the required evidence is successful completion of an examination that tests the knowledge base for the selected area of practice. Other requirements relate to the content of coursework and amount of supervised practice.

Legal Regulation

All nurses are legally accountable for actions taken in the course of professional nursing practice as well as for actions assigned by the nurse to others assisting in the provision of nursing care. Such accountability is accomplished through the legal regulatory mechanisms of licensure and criminal and civil laws.

The legal contract between society and the professions is defined by statute and by associated rules and regulations. State nurse practice acts and related legislative and regulatory initiatives serve as the explicit codification of the profession's obligation to act in the best interests of society. Nurse practice acts grant nurses the authority to practice and grant society the authority to sanction nurses who violate the norms of the profession or act in a manner that threatens the safety of the public.

Statutory definitions of nursing should be compatible with and build upon the profession's definition of its practice base, but be general enough to provide for the dynamic nature of an evolving scope of nursing practice. Society is best served when consistent definitions of the scope of nursing practice are used by states. This allows residents of all states to access the full range of nursing services.

Conclusion

Nursing's Social Policy Statement, Second Edition describes professional nursing in the United States of America. It includes an identification of the values and the social responsibility of the profession, a definition of professional nursing, a brief discussion of the scope of practice, and a description of professional nursing's knowledge base and the methods by which professional nursing is regulated. *Nursing's Social Policy Statement, Second Edition* provides both an accounting of nursing's professional stewardship and an expression of professional nursing's continuing commitment to the society it serves.

REFERENCES

1. Nursing's Agenda for the Future Steering Committee. *Nursing's Agenda for the Future* (Washington, D.C.: American Nurses Publishing, 2001). Also available on the ANA web site: http://www.nursingworld.org/naf/

2. American Nurses Association. *Nursing: A Social Policy Statement* (Kansas City, MO. American Nurses Association, 1980).

3. American Nurses Association. *Nursing's Social Policy Statement* (Washington, D.C.: American Nurses Publishing, 1995).

4. Page, B.B. "Who owns the profession?," *Hastings Center Report* 5(5): 7–8 (1975).

5. Ibid., 7.

6. Donabedian, A. Foreword in M. Phaneuf, *The Nursing Audit: Self-Regulation in Nursing Practice*, 2nd ed. (New York: Appleton-Century-Crofts, 1972), 8.

7. American Nurses Association. *Bill of Rights for Registered Nurses* (Washington, D.C.: American Nurses Publishing, 2001), 1.

8. Nightingale, F. *Notes on Nursing: What It Is and What It Is Not.* (1859; reprint, New York: J. B. Lippincott Company, 1946), preface, 75.

9. Henderson, V. *Basic Principles of Nursing Care* (London: International Council of Nurses, 1961), 42.

10. American Nurses Association, *Nursing: A Social Policy Statement.* (Kansas City, MO. American Nurses Association, 1980).

11. Adapted from: American Nurses Association. *Code of Ethics for Nurses with Interpretive Statements* (Washington, D.C.: American Nurses Publishing, 2001), 5. (Also on the ANA Web site: http://nursingworld.org/ethics/ecode.htm)

12. American Nurses Association House of Delegates. *Titling for Licensure* (Kansas City, MO: American Nurses Association, 1985).

13. American Nurses Association. *Nursing: Scope and Standards of Practice* (Washington, D.C.: American Nurses Publishing, 2003).

14. American Nurses Association, *Code of Ethics for Nurses with Interpretive Statements*, 13–14.

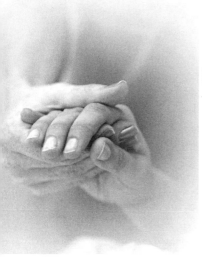

Index